Praise for *Sex Magic*

"I've trusted Dr. Laura Berman for years with advice on love, relationships, and everything in between. *Sex Magic* is like her advice on steroids—insightful, real, and transformational. Don't just read this book—live it."
—Nick Cannon, entertainer and media mogul

"If you're ready to stop playing small in your relationships, *Sex Magic* is the book for you. Dr. Laura Berman combines practical strategies with powerful insights to help you unlock the kind of intimacy that creates massive growth and transformation. This is more than a book—it's a blueprint for success in love and connection."
—Lewis Howes, *New York Times*
bestselling author of *The School of Greatness*

"Reading *Sex Magic* felt like having a conversation with a wise, funny, and supportive friend. Dr. Laura Berman's practical tools and insightful exercises make this book a powerful resource for anyone looking to rediscover the magic in their relationships—and themselves."
—Maria Menounos, television personality, actress, producer,
New York Times bestselling author, and host of popular podcast *Heal Squad*

"I love Dr. Berman's work! If your relationship has reached a point where sex feels about as exciting as doing laundry or unloading the dishwasher, Dr. Laura Berman's latest book is the much-needed guide to reigniting desire and turning intimacy into something you actually look forward to. Dr. Berman understands that each partner brings unique challenges, vulnerabilities, and experiences to the table. With her signature mix of clarity, profound insights, and practical advice you can start implementing immediately, she helps readers navigate these intricacies and build a connection that flourishes both in and out of the bedroom. Let *Sex Magic* be your road map to a love life that's not just satisfying, but also deeply aligned, and where sex never feels like yet another boring chore on your to-do list."
—Kristina Kuzmic, comedian and author of *I Can Fix This*

"Dr. Laura Berman's *Sex Magic* is a transformative guide to intimacy and soulful connection. With over 30 years of experience, Dr. Berman blends science and spirit, offering practical tools and ancient techniques to reignite passion and remove blocks to intimacy. Her step-by-step approach empowers readers to embrace vulnerability, release inhibitions, and experience profound healing. *Sex Magic* is a must-read for anyone seeking to elevate their love life and personal growth."
—Anita Moorjani, *New York Times* bestselling author of *Dying to Be Me*

"Dr. Laura Berman has created a guide that combines the practical with the mystical in *Sex Magic*. Her exercises will awaken your energy, break down barriers, and help you access the kind of connection we all deeply crave. It's a transformational resource for anyone ready to embrace their full potential."

—Sah D'Simone, trauma-informed spiritual teacher

"As a relationship therapist and teacher, I often speak to the power of embracing vulnerability and opening our hearts. In *Sex Magic*, Dr. Laura Berman takes this idea to new heights by showing us how intimacy can be a gateway to healing, transformation, and joy. Her exercises are profound, practical, and life-changing—a must-read for anyone ready to embrace the full power of love."

—Katherine Woodward Thomas, *New York Times* bestselling author of *Calling in "The One"*

"Dr. Laura Berman's *Sex Magic* is a transformative book that shows us intimacy is far more than physical—it is an energetic and spiritual experience. With profound wisdom and practical tools, she helps readers heal past wounds, release energetic blocks, and align their energy to experience love as a sacred, soulful connection. *Sex Magic* offers a path to rediscover passion, create deeper connections, and embrace intimacy as a source of healing, wholeness, and divine connection."

—Susan Grau, author of *Infinite Life, Infinite Lessons*

"Dr. Laura Berman gets it: intimacy is about more than physical connection—it's about emotional depth and energetic alignment. *Sex Magic* is packed with exercises that help you build trust, release fear, and step into the kind of relationship that feels electric. This book is for anyone ready to do the work and reap the rewards."

—Mark Groves, human connection specialist, speaker, author, coach, podcast host, and founder of Create The Love

"In *Sex Magic*, Dr. Laura Berman offers a master class in connection. Her practical tools and inspiring exercises help you navigate intimacy with clarity, confidence, and curiosity. This book is a must-read for anyone who values love, passion, and personal growth."

—Lindsay Jill Roth, author of *Romances & Practicalities*

"In *Sex Magic*, Dr. Laura Berman asks that we remain curious about the ever after. This manual is a call for us all to practice intention, thrive, and create magic beyond the infatuation phase of our relationships. A must-read. Truly a guide for us all."

—Brandi Sellerz-Jackson, author of *On Thriving*

"A masterpiece in redefining the way we can feel about sex. Dr. Laura beautifully illustrates how to embrace both meaningful and edgy sex and how to combine the two all while expressing connection and vulnerability. This is a next-level deep dive into spirituality and sexuality and how to harness your power in an authentic way. This book is a game changer."

—Craig Siegel, *Wall Street Journal* bestselling author of
The Reinvention Formula, coach, teacher,
TEDx speaker, 8-time marathoner, and investor

"In *Sex Magic*, Dr. Laura Berman offers a wealth of practical tools and insights that empower readers to transform their intimate lives. This book is a hands on guide that not only inspires but also equips you with techniques to deepen connection, ignite passion, and manifest your desires. A must-read for anyone seeking tangible steps toward spectacular intimacy and personal transformation."

—Dr. Scott Lyons, founder of The Embody Lab

"Reading *Sex Magic* feels like a wake-up call in the best way. Dr. Laura Berman challenges you to rethink intimacy, let go of inhibitions, and prioritize connection. It's honest, empowering, and exactly the kind of book I'd recommend to anyone who wants to improve their love life."

—Nick Viall, host of *The Viall Files* and author
of *Don't Text Your Ex Happy Birthday*

SEX
MAGIC

Also by Laura Berman, PhD

Quantum Love

Real Sex for Real Women

Loving Sex

It's Not Him, It's You!

Talking to Your Kids About Sex

The Book of Love

Secrets of the Sexually Satisfied Woman

The Passion Prescription

For Women Only

You're Not Crazy, You're Just Ascending

SEX MAGIC

Take Your Body, Mind, and Relationship to the Next Level with Spectacular Intimacy

LAURA BERMAN, MSW, PHD

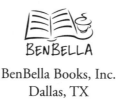

BenBella Books, Inc.
Dallas, TX

This book is for informational purposes only. The author and publisher specifically disclaim any and all liability arising directly or indirectly from the use of any information contained in this book. Any product mentioned in this book does not imply endorsement of that product by the author or publisher.

Sex Magic copyright © 2025 by Berman Institute, LLC

All rights reserved. Except in the case of brief quotations embodied in critical articles or reviews, no part of this book may be used or reproduced, stored, transmitted, or used in any manner whatsoever, including for training artificial intelligence (AI) technologies or for automated text and data mining, without prior written permission from the publisher.

BenBella Books, Inc.
8080 N. Central Expressway
Suite 1700
Dallas, TX 75206
benbellabooks.com
Send feedback to feedback@benbellabooks.com

BenBella is a federally registered trademark.

Printed in the United States of America
10 9 8 7 6 5 4 3 2 1

Library of Congress Control Number: 2024059510
ISBN 978-1-63774-694-3 (hardcover)
ISBN 978-1-63774-695-0 (electronic)

Editing by Camille Cline and Victoria Carmody
Copyediting by Amy Handy
Proofreading by Rebecca Maines and Jenny Bridges
Text design and composition by PerfecType, Nashville, TN
Cover design by Morgan Carr
Printed by Sheridan MI

Special discounts for bulk sales are available. Please contact bulkorders@benbellabooks.com.

This book is dedicated to my parents. They taught me by example about the beautiful complexities and potentials of sexuality. Along with a front-row seat to how sex can destroy relationships, they also showed me the beauty of how it can repair and create true magic.

CONTENTS

Introduction		1
CHAPTER 1	Sex Magic as a Component of Quantum Love	11
CHAPTER 2	The Ancient Wisdom of Tantra, Kundalini, and Taoism	37
CHAPTER 3	A Sex Magician's Guide to the Chakra System	63
CHAPTER 4	Erotic Embodiment for Mind-Blowing Sex	93
CHAPTER 5	The Heart as a Path to Amazing Sex	131
CHAPTER 6	Cultivating Sexual Power	155
CHAPTER 7	Leaving Inhibitions Behind	175
CHAPTER 8	Spells and Rituals for Creating Sex Magic	191
CHAPTER 9	Getting Creative with Sex Magic	217
CHAPTER 10	Pleasure for a Lifetime of Sex Magic	237
Acknowledgments		245
Appendix: Supplemental Readings		249

INTRODUCTION

As a sex, love, and relationship therapist for over thirty years, I've seen so many changes in America's bedrooms. And I'm not just talking about the fact that we now have THC-infused lubricants and sex toys that have gone from basic dildos to futuristic sex aids that can stimulate our hotspots, track our arousal, connect to our smartphones, and even steam rice. Okay, maybe not the latter, but I wouldn't be surprised if a combo vibrator/rice cooker/air fryer/ Roomba hits the market sometime soon.

What's even more important than our technological advances are the advancements in we've seen in sexual equality. Society has become more inclusive of the LGBTQIA+ community and the continuum of sexual expression. Consent and bodily autonomy have become part of our cultural lexicon. Female sexuality has been (partially) destigmatized, and female orgasms have become more prioritized. More and more people have begun to embrace the fact that gender and sexuality are fluid and multifaceted and that our romantic relationships don't need to be modeled after a 1950s sitcom.

Yet despite how much time has passed and how much has changed in the last three decades, the individuals and couples I work with have stayed the same—at least in one regard. They may have switched from flares to boot cuts to skinny jeans (and then back to flares again), but they all ask me the same question: *How can we spice things up?*

People inevitably get bored in the bedroom. Whether they are gay, straight, bi, or pan, whether they are monogamous or polyamorous, whether they are single or in a long-term relationship, people want to have the kind of sex they see in the movies. They want the kind of passion that people write songs and poems about. They want the kind of sex that almost makes their neighbors call the police to report a noise disturbance. They want the panty-ripping, sweat-dripping, forget-your-own-name kind of sex.

So they come to me, or other experts like me, and they ask: How can I make my partner more passionate? How can I have more orgasms? What toys will make our sex life more exciting? How can I last longer? How can I come harder? How can I blow his, her, or their mind when the house is a mess and the kids are whining and I haven't bought lingerie since Obama was in office (the *first* time)?

You may have seen me on television shows like *The Oprah Winfrey Show*, *The Dr. Oz Show*, or hosting my show *In the Bedroom with Dr. Laura Berman* on OWN (the Oprah Winfrey Network). Maybe you've heard me on the radio or read one of the nine books I've written. If you have, you know the advice I've often given when asked these kinds of questions. From date night ideas to sexual position tips to helping people figure out where the G-spot is or revealing whether female ejaculation is really a thing, I have spent my entire career teaching people how to have better sex and how to love and be loved better.

Most people I talk to have an almost identical idea of what sex "should" look like, from being romanced and chased to having passionate, uncomplicated sexual pleasure to wanting kisses and fireworks and the whole rom-com meets YouPorn experience. Most people I

INTRODUCTION

work with want what they have been taught, influenced, and even manipulated into wanting. These are things that line up with what we see in movies and the media—things that appear desirable and tempting, but end up being all show and no substance, and certainly not sustainable.

So many of us have begun to lose our way and fall into unconscious and addictive attitudes toward our bodies and the ways we source sexual pleasure. The truth is that you can try every sexual position under the sun. You can become an expert in oral sex techniques or have more sex toys than one of the OnlyFans stars you follow. But at the end of the day, it's still just sex. And after a while, the craziest position, role-play, or swinging encounter becomes predictable and becomes "just sex."

Don't get me wrong. "Just sex" can be pretty good. It might even be enough for some people. But if you're reading this book, it's probably not enough for you. You know that something is missing in your sex life, that there is so much more to discover. Or perhaps you sense that there are new heights you can reach in sexual pleasure and want a deep connection with your partner and yourself. You may even be aware that sexual energy is just about the highest-frequency energy our bodies can hold, and as such, it is a powerful, creative, and manifesting tool we can access and harness.

If you know what I'm talking about, if you feel the truth of this deep in your bones, then you're ready to enter the world of sex magic. You're ready to stop having "just sex," and to start *creating from* sex. You are ready to take your sex life to the next level, experiencing pleasure, mind-blowing orgasms, soul-to-soul connection, healing, and manifestation. You are ready to step into your true sexual and creative power and become the author of your own reality.

3

THE TRUE ANTIDOTE TO BEDROOM BOREDOM

We all love love, especially at the early stages, when it's all butterflies and eager anticipation. This is the stage in relationships scientists call the infatuation stage. It's a period of overwhelming intensity and we can't get enough of the feeling of it and each other. After commitment and familiarity set in, we move on to the attachment stage, which is a much softer, more sustainable kind of connection. With deeper investment and commitment comes more security and emotional connection. But for many this also brings with it less unpredictability and excitement. Without the energetic charge of discovering and capturing love, it can begin to feel boring.

This is when couples usually come to see me, often after years of lukewarm erotic connection that has led them to shut down from their intimate lives, and eventually each other, allowing a distance to build between them. By the time they enter my office, they are usually at a point of crisis. While we can't go back to those early stages of dating when we are in a long-term, committed relationship, we can absolutely create the antidote to sexual boredom. To a certain extent, this can be achieved by enhancing communication and building some spice into their relationship by exploring fantasies, role-plays, and new ways to make sex interesting.

Much of my career has been spent helping people do that. The problem is, I could give you 365 tools, toys, and role-plays to create excitement in your sexual relationship, and in a year or so you'd come back having been there, done that, and wanting more. The never-ending search for novelty is exhausting, not to mention that it often leads to all sorts of behaviors that put your relationship and even your health at risk.

INTRODUCTION

The true, *sustainable* antidote to sexual boredom is not found in exploring external ways to create novelty, but in creating and experiencing *intensity* in our sexual experience.

You don't have to stay in an infatuation stage to have soul-filling, mind-blowing intensity with your partner. Sex magic allows you to create intensity that doesn't have an expiration date. It doesn't disappear over time like the intensity of the infatuation stage does. It can last forever and actually gets better and better, as long as we are intentional about our sexual energy and how we use it.

WHAT IS SEX MAGIC?

In a world where everyone seems to be chasing stimulation and excitement in fleeting, superficial ways, sex magic is a powerful antidote—a grounded, intentional practice that reconnects us to what truly matters. It's become easy to lose touch with deeper, more fulfilling forms of intimacy and connection. Instead, in our search for spice or excitement we look in all the wrong places: porn, shallow thrills, sex outside our relationship (or that puts our relationship at risk). More often than not this leaves us feeling empty, disconnected, and craving more, as the shallow thrills fail to nourish our emotional and spiritual needs. Instead of more connection, we feel less, often even more alienated from our body and emotions.

What I call sex magic is a practice of focusing on presence over distraction, connection over escape, thrilling depth over cheap thrills, authenticity over performance, and fulfillment over emptiness. Sex magic invites us to view intimacy as sacred again. It is a practice that honors both the body and the spirit, recognizing the potential for deep emotional and even spiritual transformation that is not only emotionally satisfying but deeply erotic and physically satisfying. The sacred approach of sex magic restores a sense of reverence to the act of sex, making it a meaningful and enriching part of our lives, rather than something transactional or trivial. It is the antidote to bedroom boredom.

The philosophy and practice of sex magic, as discussed in this book, involves using ancient techniques to work with the body's energy (and that of your partner) in a conscious and intentional way. The kind of intensity we get from sex magic is based on self-revelation, vulnerability, and getting to know your partner on a soulful, intimate level. It comes from learning to play with and direct the energy of your physical arousal, to move it around you, through you, and between you. In this book, you will learn that we don't need sex swings or elaborate sex positions, although there is nothing wrong with those. Sex magic gives us the gift of never being bored with our partner or with ourselves. In fact, it's quite the opposite—it makes sex magical in the sexiest of ways!

Sex magic changes the definition of SEX to S.E.X, a Sacred Energy Exchange. That's essentially what sex is. Yes, it's physical in every sense of the word, but fundamentally sex, whether it's between you and a partner or solo, is an experience of energy moving through you and between you. And when that energy is harnessed in a conscious way, that is when sex becomes a seriously mind-blowing experience.

A NEW WAY TO LOOK AT SEXUAL ENERGY

At our core, we are all pure vibrating energy. When we interact with one another, we are communicating with so much more than just our words and our body language. Our bodies are pure atomic energy that emit an energetic frequency, a life force that lives deep within every

INTRODUCTION

living thing. Our energetic frequency shifts and changes, and we often feel it in and around us. We have all felt that crackle of energy when we've passed by someone we find attractive. We've experienced that swell of loving energy when we look at our children or wrap our arms around a friend we haven't seen for a while—that's the experience of our energetic frequency in action.

Energy especially reigns supreme in the bedroom. Do you know that tingling and warmth you feel in your genitals during arousal? That's energy. The explosion of orgasm? That's energy as well. All sexual pleasure that we exchange with our partner is an energy exchange. It's not just about the touches and strokes you share. It's about the energy behind those actions and the energy those actions create in your body. That is why you can have passionate, exciting sex with a partner you've been with for thirty years, or you can have totally boring and unsatisfying sex even with that unbelievably hot person from the bar you were eyeing all night. Energy doesn't lie. Energy can't be faked. And when we get in tune with our energy and harness that power, anything can happen—even magic.

When you engage in sex magic, your orgasmic potential is limitless. While for most people orgasms are more localized to the genital area, those who practice sex magic can have full-body sensual experiences and full-body orgasms. Once you learn how and practice moving energy around your body, the wave of orgasm can be moved through the body as well and even blow out the top of your head! You have the unfettered ability to create the most passionate, fulfilling orgasms for both you and your partner. You can even conjure and customize your orgasms to suit your mood.

Sex magic is available to us in every sexual scenario regardless of our relationship orientation or status. But our potential for experiencing sex magic exponentially increases when we are with a partner with whom we feel safe and committed. This is because couples are like human tuning forks, and we are constantly energetically "entraining" to each other. By this I mean that we automatically and almost entirely unconsciously "tune" into our partner's frequency and match it with ours. We are completely linked in the most primal and spiritual way.

Waking up to how your energy impacts your partner's energy (and vice versa) is one of the first steps in taking ownership of your sexual power and creating sex magic. It's about realizing that there is so much more to sex than just knowing the anatomy and the hot spots (although that is important too). Sex magic is about realizing what is happening on an energetic level and harnessing that power.

THE SACREDNESS OF SEX

In its purest, most perfect form, sex can be used as a tool to elevate our vibrational frequency and bring us closer to the sacred. *That is sex magic.* It is not about religion, although those from all religious backgrounds can enjoy this type of deep intimacy. Sexual arousal is one of the highest-frequency states the body can hold, yet the power we can exercise from that state is rarely discussed. Our ancestors knew this. Many Eastern philosophies and practices understand this. It's time for us to come to this primal truth again.

The idea of sexuality as a sacred path goes back millennia. It shows up in Kabbalah, Mystic Christianity, Sufism, Buddhist and Hindu Tantra, alchemy, and ceremonial magic. In Judaism, one of the most sacred acts or good deeds (mitzvah) a couple can perform is sex together. And in "The Zohar," one of the chief texts of Kabbalism, it is taught that we can use sexual union with our beloved to create a connection with God. Kabbalism teaches that sexual intimacy is one of the most powerful ways that we can create an embodied experience of God.

INTRODUCTION

The same is true in many other religions and cultures, from Christianity to paganism to Hinduism. Celebrating sexuality and being a spiritual person do not have to be mutually exclusive. But sadly, in our modern culture, we have collectively forgotten the fact that when sex is sacred it is a way to experience the highest, most blissful energies that are profound, transformational, pleasurable, and even healing.

As much as the nonphysical energies of sex will be discussed in this book, it is your beautiful body that is the true sex magic instrument. Our physical selves are not just containers for our souls. It's through our bodies that we experience the physicality of pleasurable sensations. It's in partnership with our bodies that we can harness its frequency for pleasure and magic. During the practice of sex magic, we are fully present in our bodies and with each other. This is where mind-blowing, pleasurable, intimate, and deeply satisfying sex begins!

HOW TO USE THIS BOOK

Sex Magic is intended to be a companion and guide that can be used whether you are single or in a relationship. You are going to learn brand-new things about your body, your energy systems, and how to harness and work with them in service to amazing sexual pleasure, connection, and magic.

You will learn a great deal in this book about the energetic system that is your physical body. The key to experiencing sex magic is in learning how to work with that energetic system; feel it, connect with it, move it, and share it in ways that reacquaint you with your body, energize you, and give you tremendous pleasure. So in the following pages I guide you through a variety of different exercises and tools you can practice to become a magnificent sex magician by:

SEX MAGIC

* Connecting more deeply to your body's energy
* Building the erotic energy between you and a partner
* Moving sexual energy between you and your partner
* Enhancing orgasmic intensity
* Using sex as a powerful tool to manifest your dreams

I encourage you to explore and try all of them! The exercises I share can be done alone or with a partner, but I advise you to try all the exercises alone at first. This way you can familiarize yourself with the techniques without the distraction of your partner's presence. Get comfortable with it and do any troubleshooting so that when you try it with a partner you are good to go. Get used to being a powerful, creative sexual force in your own right. Start creating some muscle memory when it comes to techniques like grounding your body's energy, shifting into heart-brain energetic coherence, and moving energy through and around your body. Doing so will make it easier for you to replicate these experiences with your partner because you will feel confident and practiced.

One last note: When it comes to trying any of these exercises with a partner, remember you can have sex magic even without your partner's active participation. They don't even need to know what you're doing. In fact, it can be really fun to experiment on them, watch their amazing response, and tell them afterward about what you did! Because of its positive intentions, sex magic cannot harm and will only help. Of course, it's ideal if you can both be on this journey together. But truthfully, if you are working at and holding the higher vibration of sex magic, your partner will automatically entrain to that energy state and begin co-creating beside you even if they don't realize it.

Get ready to begin your pleasure-filled and soul-nurturing journey to sex magic!

CHAPTER 1

Sex Magic as a Component of Quantum Love

> For one human being to love another: that is perhaps the most difficult of all our tasks, the ultimate, the last test and proof, the work for which all other work is but preparation.
>
> **—Rainer Maria Rilke**

Some people are content with "good-enough" sex. And some people are content with no sex at all. And that's okay. That's their journey. *But it doesn't have to be yours.* If you are reading this book, sex is not something secondary for you. It is not something forgettable or replaceable in your time here on this Earth. I feel that. It's not that way for me or the thousands I coach and teach either. I wrote this book for the same reason you're reading it.

I wrote this book because I believe sex can be *the most important thing we ever do with our minds, bodies, and spirits.* I believe sex is so much more than what we see in the media and what most people have come to expect and accept in the bedroom.

This is *your invitation* to stop running from your feeling of lack.

This is *your* sex magic era.

QUANTUM LOVE AND HARNESSING THE ENERGY WITHIN YOU

To understand how sexual energy can be used to bring into reality what you most desire in love and all things (known as "the art of manifestation"), we must first understand how our feelings create our reality. I summarize it here, but if you want to get into the specifics (and the science) of how this all works, and how it affects all areas of your life, definitely read my book *Quantum Love* (Hay House, 2016).

What quantum physicists have discovered in numerous studies is that our bodies' energetic frequency, when matched with (conscious or unconscious) intention, is what creates our reality. This is actually the scientific process underneath what most people know as "manifesting" or the "Law of Attraction." What sets our bodies' energetic frequency is our conscious (and unconscious) thoughts and feelings. The Latin word for emotion is *emotere*, which translates to "energy in motion." That's what emotions are; when we cry at a sad movie or yell at our partner when we feel angry, we are literally moving energy through our systems.

Our bodies' feeling states hold an energetic frequency, and different emotions have different frequencies. One of the best, most comprehensive descriptions of how this all works is found in the transformational book *Power vs. Force: The Hidden Determinants of Human Behavior* by Dr. David Hawkins (Hay House, 2014). Over twenty years, Hawkins correlated his findings (along with the findings of numerous other researchers) with thousands of patients. In the end, he was able to calibrate the relative power of the energetic frequency of different attitudes, thoughts, feelings, situations, and relationships. What he created was a consistent scale calibrating the energetic frequency of different emotional states that correlated with what psychologists, sociologists, and medical doctors could all tell you anecdotally. He called it the Map of Consciousness.

According to the Map of Consciousness, your body's energetic calibration is created by your conscious and subconscious emotional states. And it's that calibration, your body's energetic frequency, that makes you a magnet for more experiences that match those emotional states. So if you are feeling angry (consciously or even unconsciously), your body holds the energetic frequency of anger. And in that calibration of anger, you energetically attract things and experiences that reinforce your anger.

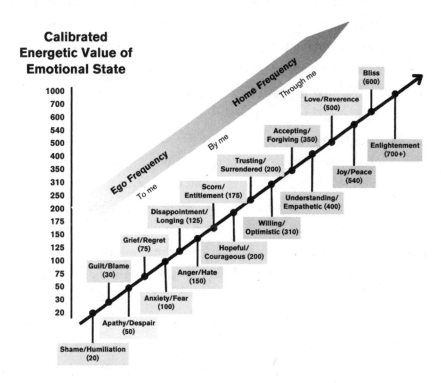

Quantum Lovemap

Just so you can get a sense of the energetic frequency your body holds in different emotional states, consider the Quantum Lovemap from *Quantum Love*, which summarizes the work of Hawkins and many others in one graph.

On the diagonal line is a series of emotional states, along with the calibration of your body's energetic frequency when in those emotional states. When your body is calibrating below a frequency of 200, you are considered to be in what I refer to on the Quantum Lovemap as "ego frequency." I often refer to this as a "To Me" state of being. You feel you aren't in the driver's seat of your life and instead experience yourself at the effect of what gets thrown at you. In ego frequency you are spending time in uncomfortable states like guilt, shame, regret, anger, and disappointment. As you move up the scale, between 200 and 400 you are in what I refer to as the "By Me" energetic frequency. This is the beginning of what I call "Home Frequency" (because it's really the natural state we are born into), and in the beginning of the Quantum Love zone. You feel more in your power and peace when you are in emotional states like hopefulness, willingness, trust, and optimism. Once you are in feeling states above a calibration of 400, like empathy, forgiveness, joy, and love, you are really humming in Home Frequency and living in what I call the "Through Me" state, fully experiencing Quantum Love.

If you want to know where you tend to live on the Quantum Lovemap, you can take the Quantum Love quiz on my website (https://drlauraberman.com/sexmagic). The main thing to know is that we rarely stay in one place on the Quantum Lovemap. And most of us rarely reach, much less stay at, a calibration of 700 or above. But the state of extreme sensual pleasure and orgasm puts us there! This is one of the keys to sex magic.

Our thoughts and feelings are vibrational energy waves—the same energy waves that exist in everything around us. Every thought you

SEX MAGIC AS A COMPONENT OF QUANTUM LOVE

have, have ever had, or will ever have creates a vibration that goes out into the quantum field, extending forever. The energy of our emotions is *manifesting* the events and relationships that occur in our lives on a quantum level. This is the defining idea behind the Law of Attraction.

The concept of "Quantum Love" is simple: We seem solid, as does everything and everyone else around us. But that is an optical illusion. If you were to look at yourself through an atomic microscope, you would see that you are pure vibrating energy.

When I use the word "energy," I don't just mean your physical energy (like feeling awake and active versus tired or worn out). Every single one of us gives off a vibration (think of it as a frequency) to the world around us.

When it comes to relationships, you and your partner are like tuning forks, matching your bodies' energetic frequencies to one another and mutually creating the tone of your relationship experience. Lower-frequency feelings like fear, shame, guilt, anger, and despair will bring more of the experiences you *don't* want to your relationship. Higher-frequency feelings like acceptance, forgiveness, joy, and elation create more of what you *do* want.

To understand what this all looks like in action, let's take a look at an example of how we create our realities on two levels, the practical 3D level and the quantum level.

Here is an example of how we create our realities on the 3D level: Your partner comes home from work in a bad mood. You instantly start to feel yourself get sucked into that same state. Maybe you're annoyed that they are being dismissive or grouchy. Maybe you're feeling like you're to blame for their bad mood or that you aren't "enough" for them. These internal scripts will happen without you even realizing it. Most of them were set into our minds before we were even old enough to understand those thoughts.

Now, a person who is working on their healing and growth might be able to throw on the brakes and start to notice these thoughts, to stay open and curious, and even to think, "What if I picked thoughts that made me feel better?" From there, an energy shift can happen. You can start to release your responsibility to control your partner's mood and to hold your own energetic space, inviting your partner to come into your peace when they are ready.

Beautiful, right? But it can go even deeper than that.

Here is an example of how we can create our realities on a quantum level. Before your partner walks through the door in a bad mood, you've already been consciously curating your day by picking and sustaining activities that feel good to your mind and body, and thoughts that serve you and your goals on this planet. You've had a busy, stressful day, one that would normally wear you out and put you in a vulnerable energetic state, but now things are different.

Things are different because:

* *You deeply believe that everything that happens to you is a potential gift.* Every experience is here to serve you, to serve your growth. Your partner's bad mood is then not just something for you to overcome, but something for you to welcome and acknowledge. It's a chance for you to practice boundaries, both in how you want to be treated and how much you are willing to let your peace be affected by anyone or anything else around you.

* *You're not comparing your relationship to any "ideal" relationship.* Your partner's bad mood doesn't feel like a punishment or an accusation that you aren't a good enough partner. It doesn't feel overwhelming or shameful, like something you need to hide from the outside world, nor take responsibility

SEX MAGIC AS A COMPONENT OF QUANTUM LOVE

for creating. You're not comparing your relationship to people you see online or in the media, or to a past version of how things used to be in your relationship.

* *You're secure not only in your relationship to your partner, but to yourself.* You can competently handle any issues in your relationship, and any storm can be weathered as long as you stay connected to each other. But most of all, you stay connected to yourself. You can't control how your partner responds, but you can control your willingness to stand for yourself with love while still keeping your heart open and compassionate to your partner's struggle.

* *You intuitively know that your partner is your soulmate.* Because of this, you will trigger each other's growth potential, meaning you will get on each other's nerves sometimes! You will also each have a unique ability to heal and mend the psychic wounds that the other carries, but *only* after you let yourself stay with the discomfort of growth.

Can you see how much differently you will experience your partner's bad mood if you're choosing to exist in the above mindset? You won't need to escape to protect yourself. You won't be swept up in the momentary painful drama of feeling "not good enough" or fearing what is happening. You will be flowing in Home Frequency.

If you are in Home Frequency, you won't be protecting your energy from your partner, but you will be powerfully influencing them to meet and match your energy, without them necessarily noticing nor you even trying!

I know, I know. It's not as easy as it sounds, but that's a good thing. It's not easy but it's possible, and *it's worth it,* and the journey to get there is the whole point of why you are here on this planet. Because once you master your own peace and hold your own frequency, everyone and everything matches *you*. Not the reverse.

THE POWER OF SEX MAGIC AND CONSCIOUS SEXUAL INTENTION

With sex magic, we not only connect with and inhabit our energetic bodies, but connect that energetic body with our sexual arousal centers and learn to create conscious energetic sexual exchanges with our partners.

Marrying the etheric/energetic body and the physical body isn't an easy task for most of us. In fact, many of us were brought up to believe that the spirit cannot partake in sensual pleasures. Maybe you were taught that sex is dirty or even that your genitals are dirty. You might have learned it was sinful to enjoy the pleasures of the flesh, and that when you *did* enjoy it, it was a sign that you were sinful and in need of forgiveness.

So much shame. A whole mountain of it. And it's standing between you and everything you ever wanted out of your sex life. (We'll get into that a little more in chapter 7.) Even if you are sexually uninhibited, you might not be able to stay present during sex. You might struggle to accept your body—let alone to revel in it and marvel at its beauty.

The truth is that our society has gone from treating sex as something taboo to treating it as something to be bought and sold, and we can see this attitude reflected in our sexual energy. There are shades of shame and impudence in our bedrooms, an almost teenage defiance that it's okay to watch porn whenever we want, even if we secretly judge ourselves for being so "needy" and being so unsatisfied all the time.

SEX MAGIC AS A COMPONENT OF QUANTUM LOVE

What you need to know is that having sex magic isn't about a *lack* of shame, but a surplus of acceptance. A wealth of intention. An overflowing of conscious, present-oriented thought. Sex magic supercharges your sensual and sexual pleasure.

We want our sex lives to be meaningful and sacred, but kinky and raw all at the same time. And I can help you get there. But the first step is to be honest about what is currently happening for you energetically when you have sex, whether it is masturbation or sex with partner(s). So let's do a deep dive into what is happening for you right now when you have sex.

Answer these questions as honestly as you can:

* What are the top three physical feelings I notice in my body during sex?
* What are the top three emotions I notice feeling during sex?
* What thoughts do I often have to avoid? What thoughts do I have to work to create?

How hard was it for you to answer those questions? Did you have to really focus to bring any of these sensations or memories to the surface? Did you think, "Wait, I can't answer these until I have sex again?"

It's understandable if you struggled, but it's also a sign that your physical body and your spiritual body aren't linked up right now. Not every sexual experience will be memorable down to the last moment, but if it all feels like a blur or if you have trouble recalling how it felt to be in your body at that moment . . . then you weren't.

You weren't in your body. You were somewhere else stuck in your mind, and as a result you might have had an orgasm, but it won't be anything like the kind of orgasms you can have when you practice sex magic, when your whole self is embodied and present and consciously participating.

Consciousness is the very first step in bridging the gap between your physical body and energetic body. And this is something you can start doing right now. Whether you are single or in a long-term relationship, you can start training yourself to bring consciousness to your physical sensations. Over time, you will find that you won't have to "work" so hard at this practice and that paying attention to your body's physical experiences will become second nature.

Chapter 4 explores strategies for erotic embodiment in depth. For now, I encourage you to explore the following activities that will help you bring your physical self in closer communion with your quantum self and energetic body.

Name the Physical Sensations

Start using physical sensations to describe your mood. For instance, instead of saying, "I am so anxious right now," you might observe, "My stomach feels heavy and tight. My hands are trembling, and I can't take a deep breath."

This will help you to realize that so much of what we experience on the inside is directly linked to what is happening on the outside. You will stop seeing your moods as something that just "happens" to you, but rather as transitory experiences that you can feel physically and emotionally. In addition, identifying your physical emotions will empower you to take charge of what is happening to you. Instead of feeling like a hapless victim who has no control over your mood, you will realize that you do have some choices.

Now, instead of thinking, "I am aroused," or "I want to have sex right now," you will begin instead to realize, "I feel warmth and energy spreading to my genitals," or "My heart is racing and I feel like I'm on a roller coaster," or "My nipples feel tight and super-sensitive."

SEX MAGIC AS A COMPONENT OF QUANTUM LOVE

Noticing these physical experiences is part of becoming embodied in the bedroom, and a key part of conscious sexual intention.

And here's a bonus: If you are someone who has ever struggled with "dirty" talk in the bedroom or with sending sexy texts, simply stating your physical experiences like the above examples is a great place to start! That's right, you don't have to be a Sensual Shakespeare to be a natural at erotic talk. Just share what is happening for you, like "I get so hard when I think about fucking you," or "I get butterflies when you kiss me like that."

Invite Your Physical Self to Your Day

This sounds weird, I know. You might be thinking, "Um, my physical self is already with me all day. I'm not a ghost!"

But I bet if you spend a few minutes thinking about it, you will realize that isn't true. How many times have you eaten so much that you didn't feel good, or you were so busy that you forgot to eat? How many times have you stayed up late binging your favorite series or doomscrolling on your smartphone instead of going to sleep? How many times have you given yourself a headache by drinking too much coffee, or a hangover from drinking too much alcohol?

In all of these events, there is proof that you have, at least temporarily, abandoned your physical body. Yes, I am sorry to say it, but all those times you ate a handful of candy for breakfast, you were abandoning your body. All those times you forced your tired eyes open because you couldn't or didn't want to go to bed? Body abandonment. All those times you chugged coffee instead of drinking water and going for an energetic walk? Body abandonment.

And yes, all those times you had sex while mentally thumbing through your to-do list or all those times you had sex when you didn't really want to or all those times you had sex when you faked an orgasm or all those times you were too drunk or distracted to even really pay attention were body abandonment.

I'm not telling you this to make you feel bad. This happens to everyone, especially in our hectic modern lifestyles. You almost *have* to abandon your physical needs sometimes, like when you're taking care of a newborn, or you're traveling, or you're on a major deadline and you can't stop for lunch.

But that just makes it all the more meaningful and important when we do invite our bodies to participate in our day. That's why something as simple as a thirty-minute yoga routine can have a lingering positive impact long after we put away our mats. Anytime we can connect with our bodies and give them some TLC, we are going to reap the benefits.

Exercise is a great way to get embodied. Most of us need to experiment a bit in order to find out what type of exercise best suits our body-mind connection. For instance, I personally don't feel embodied when I am running. It's too intense for me to slow down and *feel* my body, but if you're a lifelong runner who gets in that zone while running, then that works for you. For me, yoga, hiking, walking my dogs, and dancing (sometimes two at the same time!) are my go-tos for exercise that gets my body moving and awakens my awareness to my physical self.

Another added benefit of exercise is that as you awaken to your body, you're going to suddenly realize, "wait, I'm really thirsty right now," or "wow, this spending time in Savasana during yoga class was the first time that I have really taken a deep breath all day." It's like your body has been screaming quietly at you for hours, but because it's so used to you not listening to it, it just cried itself to sleep and gave up.

SEX MAGIC AS A COMPONENT OF QUANTUM LOVE

Inviting movement gives us an opportunity to pause and let our body be heard, whether it's "Stretch me here; I have blocked energy in my chest," or "Let me dance this out; I need to move!" Once you start making a habit of listening to your body while you exercise, you will find you begin to do it throughout the day more readily. You will be more likely to reach for spring water instead of a soda, or to go to sleep and let Netflix wait for the weekend.

You can also start connecting your physical body to your energetic body by paying attention to the sensualness of everyday life. You might not realize it, but your whole day is filled with delights for the senses. Start interacting with the world without taking it for granted. Notice the warm, enveloping drops of water when you stand in your shower. What parts of your body feel it the most? Is it your scalp, your backside, your hands? Feel the way the soap suds slip through your fingers. Feel the hard porcelain under your bare feet, the touch of metal on your hands when you make the water warmer.

Now, I don't expect you to get twitterpated every time you have to do a household chore. But I am simply showing you that when we start noticing our physical senses and naming those feelings, it's an immediate pathway to building that connection between our bodies and our spirits.

The senses are sacred. They have messages for you. They are waiting to be attended to, finally, after all this time. When you start doing that, even if it's only for thirty seconds at a time when you notice, "Oh my gosh, the breeze smells so good" or the slight pause you give to a birdsong that makes you smile, you're starting to build those neural connections. You're starting to rewire your brain and make pathways for more of these thoughts in the future. And the more pathways you make, the faster and more readily these thoughts will be able to spring forth. You won't have to *try* to notice the warmth of your mug of coffee. You won't have to put effort into realizing how good it feels to walk barefoot in the dewy morning grass.

This will all automatically begin to translate to you being more embodied in the bedroom and to being more sexually conscious. The next time you're having sex, challenge yourself to pay attention to what is going on with every part of your body, whether it's the way your toes slightly curl or the way your mouth parts or the way you feel spent and satiated afterward.

If it's too much to focus on just everything at once, pick just one body part to really focus on, like "I am going to pay attention to what happens to my breasts during sex," or "I want to notice how my heartbeat changes during sex."

You can also do this for everyday activities like cuddling, kissing, hand-holding, and more. And if these aren't everyday activities for you, that's okay. Start experimenting with how it would feel physically if you kissed your partner before work every morning. Notice what sensations come up for you, and how those sensations alter your day.

Now, the next time you have sex or masturbate, go back and try to answer those three questions I asked you earlier in this chapter. How quickly do the answers come to you? Are you surprised at how easy it was to source physical memories and recall exactly how you felt? That's the result of your strengthened physical and emotional connection. Congratulations! You're taking strong steps to becoming embodied and being *right here, right now,* especially during sex.

CONNECTING TO YOUR ENERGETIC BODY

You've now begun to build a connection to your physical body. Now it's time to start building awareness of and connecting to your energetic

SEX MAGIC AS A COMPONENT OF QUANTUM LOVE

body. When I talk about the energetic body, I am referring to two aspects: the subtle energetic pulses and frequencies running through (and ultimately between) our bodies, as well as our spiritual selves.

The subtle energetic vibrations and rhythms that run through the body are often described as the underlying currents of life-force energy, which animate and sustain our physical, emotional, and mental well-being. While they may not be easily perceivable through the five senses, many spiritual and holistic traditions believe in the existence of these subtle energies and their profound influence on our health and consciousness.

One common explanation for these subtle energetic vibrations is rooted in Eastern philosophies such as Hinduism, Buddhism, and Taoism, which describe a system of energy channels (nadis), energy centers (chakras), and vital breath (prana or qi) that circulate throughout the body. According to these traditions, disruptions or imbalances in the flow of energy can lead to physical illness, emotional disturbances, and spiritual disconnection. (For more details on these traditions, see chapter 3.)

Recent advancements in fields such as biofield science and psychophysiology have begun to shed light on the subtle energetic dynamics of the body. Research suggests that the human body emits bioelectromagnetic fields that interact with the surrounding environment and may play a role in regulating physiological processes.

Part of the fun of sex magic begins when we can start to sense, tap into, and play with the subtle energies running through and around our bodies, which you will do when practicing the exercises I present in this book. Sensing and playing with the energetic frequency of the body involves developing the ability to perceive and interact with the subtle vibrations and rhythms that underlie physical, emotional, and mental states.

As you make your way through this book, you will continue to explore different aspects of sensing, moving, and playing with the body's energy. But for now, here are some other ways to begin tapping into and sensing your body's energy:

* **Body awareness**: Begin by bringing your attention to your own body. Notice any sensations, tensions, or areas of discomfort. Pay attention to the quality of energy in different parts of your body. Try to notice subtle shifts in temperature, tingling sensations, or areas of increased or decreased flow.

* **Visualization:** Engage in visualization practices to play with the energetic frequency of your body. Where attention goes, energy flows. Imagine light flowing into the top of your head and filling your body. Imagine it pooling in the center of your chest and growing more intense and vibrant with every breath. Imagine the light getting so big it expands out of you all around you so you are surrounded by a field of vibrant, pulsating energy. Visualize this energy expanding and contracting with each breath, filling your entire being with light and vitality. Imagine it running up and down your system. Notice if you can sense the subtle sensations.

* **Movement or dance:** Move your body freely and intuitively to music or rhythm. Allow yourself to express and release any stagnant energy or tension through movement. Even better, make it a point to move your hips in non-linear, even figure-eight patterns. This not only loosens the hips for better flexibility during sex, but it keeps the energy moving in that area. Pay attention to how different movements and gestures affect your energy and mood.

SEX MAGIC AS A COMPONENT OF QUANTUM LOVE

* **Sound bathing:** Experiment with sound vibrations to harmonize and balance your energy body. Use or listen to instruments such as singing bowls, tuning forks, or drums to create frequencies that resonate with your own energetic field. Notice how different sounds and frequencies feel in and around your body, and how they affect your state of being.

* **Energy healing:** Seek out guidance from experienced energy healers or practitioners who can help you explore and develop your sensitivity to subtle energy. Receive energy healing sessions to experience firsthand how skilled practitioners work with the energetic frequency of the body to promote healing and balance.

THE ENERGY OF OUR SPIRIT SELVES

Sex magic at its finest does not just work with the energy of our physical bodies, but also the energy of our spiritual selves as well. When I refer to our spiritual selves, I am referring to our essential selves.

What is the essential self? Buddhist monk, writer, and teacher Thich Nhât Hanh refers to the image of a mountain and says that we are, at our very essence (or in our essential selves), the *inside* of the mountain. All kinds of chaos can happen on the mountain's surface. There can be huge storms, mudslides, or avalanches. But the inside of the mountain is unaffected and doesn't change. Your essential self is the inside of your mountain. It is eternally perfect, strong, and brilliantly radiating light in your optimal frequency.

There's a simple way to experience your essential self. Sit quietly and close your eyes. Then silently in your mind, say hello to yourself. The one who is saying hello is your personality self, the mind. The one who is listening to or *hears* "hello" is your eternal, true essential self.

The most important thing to remember is that quantum physics has proven that this energy can never be created or destroyed. It can only be transferred or transformed. Your energetic self is the part of you that will live forever. It will not always live in this body, but it can never be destroyed or diminished. It is your impenetrable life force, and it is *you*.

It is more you than anything else about you. It is more you than your birthmark. It is more you than your freckles. It is more you than the lips you inherited from your mother. It is more you than the scar from your car accident, or your fingerprints, or your eye color. It is the part of you that existed before you were on this Earth and the part of you that will exist after you leave this Earth. This is your body's energy, or what I like to call your energetic awareness.

Working with your body's energy is the key to the most amazing, mind-blowing, powerful sex you're ever going to have, yet for most of us, it's just a witness, not a participant. Learning not only to identify but also to bring awareness of your body's energy into the bedroom is a life-changing way to forever elevate your sexual experiences.

The truth is that bringing energetic awareness into the bedroom is not as straightforward as bringing your attention to your physical body. It's not about following the sensual clues that your physical body gives. But it's simpler than you think. The following section provides you with a taste of what it's like to work with your body's energy in a way you can feel. The first place to start is with what I call the grounding meditation. What you are doing during the grounding meditation is coming back into your body; inhabiting it fully. It's a key technique that you will use repeatedly when initiating some of the techniques you are going to learn to practice sex magic.

Grounding Meditation

You can listen to a guided version of this mediation at drlauraberman .com/sexmagic.

1. Sit or stand in a comfortable position. It works even better when you can be barefoot on the ground or grass.
2. Close your eyes and take some deep, slow breaths; in through the nose and out through the mouth
3. As you slowly breathe in, imagine a beautiful, brilliant light streaming into your body through the top of your head. As you slowly inhale, imagine that light (any color that occurs to you) filling every cell. Perhaps hold your breath for a beat while you imagine the light filling every corner of your body.
4. As you breathe out slowly, imagine that light shooting out your tailbone deep into the earth, making roots there.
5. Take five breaths like this, with the light flowing in through the top of your head and filling your body, and as you breathe out, letting it shoot out your tailbone deep into the earth, grounding you there.

Once you have completed the five grounding breaths, keep your eyes closed for a minute. How do you feel? You probably feel a little calmer than you did before. You also may feel some heaviness in your hips or other parts of your body. This is what it feels like to energetically inhabit your body! If you're willing, I encourage you to ground as much as possible throughout the day. Put up sticky notes around your house or in your car that say "Ground" or set an alert on your smartphone to go off every several hours. And when reminded, go through the steps above. You will find you are more tapped in and tuned in, have greater access to your intuition, and primed to dive into sex magic as you learn the techniques shared throughout this book.

For now, I encourage you to continually ground yourself in your body. Then practice connecting to that energetic body by listening to your thoughts. Now, you might think, how can I listen to my thoughts while I'm thinking them? Because you have an energetic body! You have a built-in witness who is always listening. You're just too distracted and busy to notice it noticing you.

So make a conscious effort to pull up an internal seat. Watch your waves of thoughts come in and out like tides. Don't attach yourself to the thoughts or let yourself make judgments about them. That is not the role of the energetic body. Judgment doesn't exist for the energetic body. Does the sky judge the clouds, or the stars? Does a tree judge its branches or the birds who nest in it?

No. Neither can your energetic mind judge your thoughts or your behavior. There is nothing you are doing "wrong" at this moment. There is nothing to fix. Nothing to perfect. Nothing to control. You are purely existing and noticing that existence. Feeling the fullness of each moment and considering it with curiosity.

Start making time for this practice every day. It will only take a few moments. Maybe even try building it into your day, such as when you're on the bus or waiting at the grocery store or sitting on your yoga mat. Build up your tolerance for noticing without judgment. (It may feel intolerable at first, because boy, do we humans like to judge!)

Your body is pure atomic energy. To practice sex magic, you must learn to sense the subtle (and often not so subtle) energies of your body and work with them. The exercises in this chapter will further teach you how to begin to connect with and harness those energies. They will also assist you in becoming more embodied, which is fundamental to experiencing maximum pleasure (more on this in chapter 4). When you are in your body, you are in your full power. These exercises will help you come home to your body and fully inhabit your physical form.

Tapping into your body's energy

You've already learned that you are pure energy. You've learned to ground that energy. Here's an exercise to help you start feeling the energetic signature of your body and maybe even the bodies of others as you practice:

1. Start by grounding yourself as you learned in the preceding section.

2. Rub the palms of your hands together briskly for fifteen to thirty seconds. Then gently and slowly pull your palms apart. Move your palms slightly toward and away from each other; almost like you are clapping without the palms actually meeting. Focus on what you feel between your palms. You may feel density or static; this is energy. Play with this sensation for a moment, pulling your hands a little farther apart and closer together.

3. Now let's see if you can feel the energy between your palm and the skin of your arm. This works best on bare skin, so if you need to, roll up your sleeve. Once you've rubbed your palms together again for fifteen to thirty seconds, place one palm as close as possible, hovering over your bare forearm, but not touching it. Gently run your palm up and down, hovering over the bare skin. Can you feel the same static and density between your palm and arm? This is your body's energy being felt. Some would say it's your aura. You can practice pulling your palm a little farther away, and then closer to your forearm. You can also practice this on other parts of your body.

SEX MAGIC

Note: If you'd like to take this exercise to a sensual or sexual level, practice the same technique, but instead hover your hand(s) over your genitals or other erogenous zones. Notice what you feel. Then, with your partner's permission, you can try it on their genitals.

Seeing Your Aura

Can you sense and see your aura? The aura is the energy field surrounding your entire body and has been demonstrated in numerous experiments (although scientists call it the biofield).

Auras even have colors and have not only been featured in religious paintings, but also described in numerous healing traditions. I have found that it is easier to see the aura itself than to discern its color, but we certainly are capable of both! Here's how you do it:

1. First, make sure you are grounded. It helps to be in a quiet place with dim light.
2. You can ask a partner or friend to help you practice. It's easiest to learn to see someone's aura if they are sitting still in front of a neutral background. You can even choose a sleeping pet, or someone sitting still at a coffee shop or on the bus. If you don't have another living being to practice with, you can even do this with your hand or foot. As you master this, you will be able to practice with people in movement.
3. Stare at your subject and soften your gaze as you do, almost as you might do while daydreaming. You are staring, but not focused on the details, almost staring through them.
4. After a moment, put your softened gaze on the edge of the object you are observing. If you are staring at a person, place your softened gaze right above the top of their head at first, almost like you are staring past them.

5. See if you can recognize a blurry field around the edges of the object or individual of your focus. It almost looks like the blurry field that heat radiating off asphalt in the summer might create. Usually at first you won't see any movement in this blurry field, but if you keep your gaze softened and keep practicing, you likely will see it start to undulate and move.

6. The next step once you have been able to see the aura (and maybe even perceive its moving vibration) is to see if you can sense or see the color of the aura you are observing. Remember that for most of us, the color is very subtle. At first it may just be a sense of a color. Keep practicing and it will get easier and easier.

Practice regularly and learn to trust your perception. Like any skill, seeing auras improves with consistent practice. Dedicate time to practicing in a relaxed and focused manner. The more you practice, the more attuned you may become to subtle energy fields. It can help to keep notes in a journal. Record your experiences, including any colors, sensations, or emotions you associate with auras. This can help you track your progress and gain a better understanding of how your body holds different energetic frequencies.

SEX MAGIC CASE FILE

When married couple Payal and Melissa came to see me one late August afternoon, the first thing I noticed was how bonded they seemed. Although they had only been married for three years, they had been together on and off for more than ten years.

I was curious to hear what issues could be troubling them, because they seemed so in sync, as though they truly enjoyed each other's company.

I didn't have to wait long.

"I'm weird about sex," announced Melissa with little prompting. "I can't enjoy it unless I'm drunk. I'm so inhibited, which is weird . . . because otherwise, me and her are so close. I never feel awkward being vulnerable around her, except in the bedroom."

Melissa and Payal had been in a partying mode for several years, which had hidden Melissa's awkwardness about sex. But now that they were older and had cut back on drinking, they were struggling to make sense of each other in the bedroom.

"I have started to dread initiating sex," said Payal. "I know she loves me and is attracted to me, but sex stresses her out so much that it's upsetting. I can see her mind going a million miles a minute. Now I'm starting to realize why our date nights always included several glasses of wine before we went to bed."

Over the next several weeks, I worked with Melissa one on one to source some of the stories that were causing her pain in the bedroom. I came to understand that Melissa felt like a "fraud" because Payal was her only female partner, and because she still had a lot of hidden shame about being with a woman.

"Payal is a 'gold-star lesbian,'" said Melissa. "She's only ever been with women, even in high school. Her whole family is super liberal and accepting. She's been out to them since she was nineteen years old. But I hid Payal from my family for five years . . . I mean, my parents are Mormon, for gosh sakes!

"No one from my side came to the wedding," Melissa continued, choking back tears. "I feel accepted and adored by Payal and her family, but it's not the same, y'know? I think that's why I always drank so much the last few years. I wanted to escape that pain and loneliness."

Melissa and I definitely needed to work on the shame and loss that were complicating her sexual pleasure. But while this was going to be a much longer process, I could help Melissa start to experience

SEX MAGIC AS A COMPONENT OF QUANTUM LOVE

her sexual exchanges with Payal differently in the short term. To do so I engaged Melissa in a thought experiment and guided visualization: What if, even for just one sexual encounter, she suspended all external context and all judgment? I instructed her to create a beautiful, fully judgment-free energetic vacuum, just for that one sexual encounter. There she could be with Payal and forget about her family and society. In that vacuum, there is nothing but complete acceptance and open-hearted adoration. I helped her tune into how it would feel in her body if she adored and accepted herself. Quantum love (and sex magic) does not require you to untangle painful thoughts and heal every broken place within you. Instead, it begins when we start inviting more aligned and supportive perspective and feelings into our system, and living in our bodies as though that reality already exists. Furthermore, the brain and the body don't know the difference between reality and rehearsal. So when we use our imagination to put ourselves in desired scenarios as if they are happening right here, right now, our bodies respond as if it's the truth and match that imagined scenario on a physical and energetic level.

So how would it physically feel for Melissa to feel wholeness, to feel as though she was perfectly made and perfectly accepted and supported by the universe?

She really struggled to think of a time when she ever felt that way, so she had to use her imagination. Over the next several sessions, we worked on her getting "into" her body and conjuring that feeling of wholeness on command. I knew there were times she was definitely thinking, "What does this have to do with sex?" but she trusted the process. I needed her to rewire her brain and start building neurological connections that involved positive stories about herself and her sexuality.

Unpacking the level of self-hatred Melissa struggled with would take more than a Pride march. She had to be willing to get angry at her parents (which was very difficult for this "good girl" who so desperately craved approval, especially from Mom and Dad). But all of this came secondary to her intentional practice of stepping into herself and actively beginning to conjure those feelings of wholeness and acceptance that she had denied herself since childhood. Watching her transformation was inspiring, as I saw that the happy-go-lucky, jovial person I met on our first session was just one small aspect of Melissa. Underneath that charming demeanor was someone inquisitive, challenging, and complicated, someone with a lot more power than she ever gave herself credit for.

Sexually, Melissa and Payal both started to notice changes. Payal said that Melissa started initiating sex, and that she became much more focused and less "distanced."

"She used to close her eyes and keep her face toward the pillow," said Payal. "Now she will look me deep in the eye during intimacy. It's wild how much that turns me on!"

Melissa said the change began when she realized how heavy her self-loathing was to carry and that it was a conscious choice to do so. "When I visualized how it felt to be whole and accepted, it felt so *light*. I never realized how much trauma I was carrying all the time, how much baggage I was lugging around that wasn't even all mine," she said. "When I feel that shame or embarrassment coming up, especially in the bedroom, I remember it's not mine and I can choose not to carry it. I connect to that feeling of lightness. I can feel an energetic change inside of me, like I am dropping my mask and coming out of the darkness."

This is what I love about sex magic: One tiny change can set off a chain reaction that will unlock a new world of pleasure and connection.

CHAPTER 2

The Ancient Wisdom of Tantra, Kundalini, and Taoism

What's the use of falling in love if you both remain inertly as-you-were?

—Mary McCarthy

There is such a wealth of ancient wisdom about energy and how that energy exchange works in sexual partnerships that I believe our ancestors might have been having much better sex than we are! Even though they didn't have access to expensive lingerie, warming lubrication, and electronic sex toys, they had access to knowledge about Tantra, Taoism, and Kundalini philosophies, all of which helped to make their sex lives fulfilling and fruitful.

But somewhere along the way, we lost this wealth of knowledge, especially in the Western world. Sexuality became transactional and heavily proscribed by patriarchal systems, and we stopped talking about sexual pleasure as something men and women created and rather as something shameful.

In this chapter, we explore these traditions, and I provide you with some beautiful exercises to help you begin experiencing their magic. You certainly don't have to practice these exercises every single time you have sex to enjoy the benefits. Sometimes you will only have time for a "quickie" and Tantric positions won't be on the menu. That's okay. These practices are about more than just having a twenty-four-hour orgasm (although that is a worthy goal). They are philosophies that will help you reclaim your power and purpose in the bedroom.

EXPANDING YOUR AROUSAL WITH TANTRA

Tantric texts extend all the way back to 500 CE. That is over 1,500 years ago. The philosophy began in India, although it expanded across the globe over time. Like all schools of revolutionary thought, Tantra began on the fringes. It originated among Hindus who were devotees of the god Shiva, who is one of the divine trinity in Hinduism.

Tantra is a spiritual and meditative practice that combines physical intimacy with mindfulness and deep emotional connection. The goal of Tantric sex is not only sexual pleasure but also a sense of unity, healing, and higher consciousness between partners.

The word *Tantra* has a few different meanings that apply to our erotic experience in beautiful ways. One definition is "thread" or "weave." Every time you and your partner "weave" together sexually, you are a creator sitting at a loom. You are weaving together your bodies and your energies. And together you get to weave whatever creation you desire. This is true not only during sex but during all your interactions with your partner.

Another definition of Tantra is "expansion." Tantra teaches us to expand the energies in our bodies, enhancing arousal and deepening our sensual and erotic experience. Tantra teaches us to expand our awareness of the sensual energies moving within and between us. We can also think of expansion in a physical sense. During sex, blood flow increases to our genitals. Our veins expand with this pulsing blood flow, with this Shiva force. Both males and females experience an expansion during sex. In males, this presents as an erection and as a heaviness in the testicles. In females, this presents as an engorged clitoris and even visibly enlarged labia.

As our physical form expands, Tantric sex invites us to expand in awareness inside our bodies and our souls as well. Our bodies are giving us the clues: Sex isn't about turning inward or growing smaller, sticking to a tightly constrained path with prescribed roles and behaviors. We are invited to weave new threads and expand in ever widening circles of creation.

And finally, Tantra means "liberation," which is the ultimate goal of Hinduism. Achieving liberation means to be saved from the cycle of "samsara," the cycle of birth, suffering, and death. It means you are no longer living in a world of delusion but a world of complete oneness.

In Tantric sex, intercourse can be used as a way to get that much closer to liberation and divinity. Sex becomes an opportunity to move closer to your God-self and closer to your partner's God-self. It brings you that much closer to escaping samsara, and liberating yourselves from the chains of ordinary existence.

Soul Gazing

One of my favorite Tantric exercises for enhancing and deepening intimacy in couples is soul gazing. Soul gazing can help you create powerful intimacy between you and your partner and allow for deeper bonds than you could have ever reached otherwise. It sets the stage for a connected and a magical sex experience.

While you are doing this exercise there should be no talking. You can do soul gazing on its own or utilize it as part of (or even preceding) foreplay to get completely present and connected on every level. You can soul gaze with your partner while fully clothed, but it's even better when you are fully undressed. It's a powerful exercise to try during sex as well. (If you don't have a partner, guess who you can soul gaze with? That's right, yourself in a mirror!)

Ideally soul gazing should last at least two minutes. This will actually feel like a *very* long time when starting out. It's totally normal to feel uncomfortable at first when trying soul gazing, mostly because it is so intimate. If you feel awkward or giggle a little bit, feel free to get the giggles out, but then come back to it. This is just nervousness rooted in how unaccustomed you are to the deep intimacy soul gazing delivers. I can promise if you stay with it, the awkwardness will pass and the magic will kick in.

1. Sit facing one another on the bed or some other soft surface. You can support yourself any way you wish with pillows or a headboard. I love recommending soul gazing in the Tantric position called Yab Yum. This is where the larger partner sits cross-legged or with legs extended and back supported, and the smaller partner sits on their lap facing their partner, wrapping their legs around their partner's waist, and supported by their embrace.

2. Take a moment to ground yourselves (teach your partner if they don't know how). Just this will take your connection in your daily life to a beautiful new level, not to mention that it will help resolve any arguments more quickly!

3. Next, each of you places your right hand over your partner's heart. Put your awareness on your partner's heartbeat. See if

you can feel the thumping of their heart as you imagine your heartbeats synchronizing, matching one another.

4. As you keep your hand over your partner's heart, begin to stare deeply into their left eye (directly above the heart). As you do so, imagine you are communicating and sending love or passion into your partner's eyes. Visualize the energy traveling through your partner's entire body.

5. Now begin to synchronize your breath. Take slow, deep, gentle breaths while continuing to gaze into your partner's left eye. Keep your face, mouth, and jaw relaxed. Let the back of your throat relax.

6. Try to make your breath a continuous circle. Stare into your partner's eyes and breathe the circular breath into each other's mouths.

Soul gazing during sexual exchanges makes the experience so much richer and deeper. It also slows things down in a beautiful way. After you have mastered soul gazing during foreplay, I encourage you to try it during intercourse, any time you are in a position that is face to face. Just stay perfectly still during soul gazing and then begin movement if you wish. You will find it intensifies the experience and creates even more arousal.

The Tantric Triple Lock

This is an extremely powerful Tantric exercise that you can do with a partner or on your own. It draws energy from the top of the body down to the pelvis. This can build sexual energy because it directs your chi (life force or life energy in the Tantric tradition) to your pelvic area (your root and sacral chakras) and your genitals. (You'll learn all about the chakras in chapter 3.)

The three "locks" you will be accessing and contracting are the neck, abdominal, and anal muscles, in a key order at key times. The first step is to just sit comfortably with your back and shoulders straight and supported. Hold your head upright, looking straight ahead, and then proceed with the following steps:

1. First comes throat lock. Pull your chin toward your chest, like you are pinching a pencil between your chin and neck. Hold this for a count of three, then slowly relax, raising your head. Take a deep breath in through the nose, out through the mouth.

2. Next is the abdominal lock. Draw your abdomen in, as if you are trying to touch your spine with your belly button. Tighten your abdominal muscles as you do so. Hold for a count of three, then release. Take a deep breath in through the nose, out through the mouth.

3. The anal lock is last and just involves contracting the muscles that you would use if you were holding in a bowel movement. Squeeze and hold your anus tightly, and then squeeze more firmly still. Hold this tightest squeeze for a count of three, and then relax. Again, take a deep breath in through the nose and out through the mouth.

Once you've practiced how to access each of the locks, it's time to try to squeeze them all at the same time, without releasing the previous locks. Squeeze the throat, and keep it squeezed while you add in your abdominals, and as those two areas stay contracted, add in the anal lock. According to Tantric experts and teachers, this draws the energy downward.

THE ANCIENT WISDOM OF TANTRA, KUNDALINI, AND TAOISM

Once you have mastered the triple lock, coordinate it to your breath, which is key for moving sexual energy through you. Begin by breathing out fully and slowly. Take a deep breath in and imagine your belly filling up. Now close the locks, working top to bottom, hold your breath as long as you can, and then exhale.

Are you ready to deepen and intensify your orgasm? Once you've practiced the triple lock system on your own first, without sexual stimulation, you can practice during self-stimulation or with a partner. Just move into the triple lock just as you feel your orgasm approaching and you will see how much more pleasurable and intense the experience becomes!

AROUSING YOUR KUNDALINI

Kundalini is part of Tantric philosophy. While Shiva is the creative, pulsing life force associated with Tantra, within that world exists the Hindu goddess Shakti. Shakti is the divine feminine. But Shakti is not lesser than Shiva, nor is she his opposite. They are united and inseparable, and each of them exists because of the other, as well as inside, outside, and all around each other. Separating Shakti from Shiva is like separating a mote of sunlight from the Sun itself. It's impossible.

But they interact with the world in differing ways. Shakti is often depicted as a resting, coiled-up snake, known to many as the Kundalini snake. She lives below the sacral chakra (at the base of the spine) and her latent energy emanates throughout the higher body.

Shakti's energy is latent and resting but not powerless. A resting snake is no less deadly than an awakened snake. But their energy and power work differently. An active, aggressive snake interacts with the world differently than a coiled-up snake that is resting and healing itself.

In the Kundalini practice, the snake encompasses sexual energy and is seen as a potent form of life force, or *prana*. When harnessed and circulated intentionally, it can awaken the snake, the Kundalini energy. Sexual energy is used not just for physical pleasure but as a means of spiritual awakening. One of the goals of practicing Kundalini is to awaken this energy and allow it to rise through the chakras (energy centers) along the spine, ultimately reaching the crown chakra, which leads to a heightened state of spiritual awareness or enlightenment. In the context of Kundalini, orgasm isn't just a physical release; it's seen as a moment where one can touch the divine. When combined with Kundalini practices, the release of energy during orgasm can merge the physical with the spiritual, offering a glimpse of oneness with the universe.

As I mentioned, Shakti lives below the sacral chakra. In women, this can be found at the cervix, which is located in the vagina at the base of the uterus. In men, this energy is housed at the perineum, the area between the testes and anus.

Learning to arouse Kundalini means that we assist and allow the coiled snake to slowly unravel, raising itself up through our bodies and beyond our third eye. It's important not to take the representation of the snake too lightly. The snake's body and position are very meaningful.

In the Kundalini tradition, the serpent is not asleep or just resting. It is coiled up in a protective position, and it is often shown as protecting a gem or something else priceless. The gem was sometimes referred as *Mani* or *Naagmani,* which means the jewel of the cobra. In this case, when you raise Kundalini, you discover this jewel, which is awareness. Once Kundalini has become aroused, you keep that jewel forever because a person who is enlightened cannot become unenlightened.

THE ANCIENT WISDOM OF TANTRA, KUNDALINI, AND TAOISM

That is why Kundalini should not be approached lightly. Some say that their Kundalini arousal created complete upheaval in their entire lives. Once you achieve this state, you must expect that you may need to rewrite your story in many ways. You might find yourself called upon to change careers or move countries. You might change your relationships or your spiritual practices. The arousal of Kundalini must be approached with thoughtfulness and solemnity, as one would approach a temple or a place of holy importance, because that is exactly what you are doing. But this temple lives internally and can only be seen with your inner self.

There are many ways to arouse Kundalini. These include yoga, breathwork, meditation, and kriyas. Kriyas can be translated from the Sanskrit to mean "a completed action" or a "whole action," and it refers to any set of practices that is performed with a specific goal. For instance, if you wanted to focus on arousing sexual energy, you would perform a Kriya with that goal in mind, and you might do a set of breathwork and yoga.

Kundalini Breathing Exercise

Here's a beautiful exercise for enhancing intimacy and beginning to step into the beautiful energy exchange that sex can provide. Sit unclothed with your partner on a soft but supportive surface. If you prefer not to be fully undressed, you can wear light, unrestrictive clothing.

1. Sit in the Yab Yum position described earlier (larger partner sits with back supported and smaller partner sits on their lap, facing them, legs wrapped around their torso). The smaller partner can place their hands on the larger partner's shoulders

so that you can maintain comfortable eye contact, with your faces close together.

2. If you can, maintain eye contact

3. Now breathe in deeply, picturing your breath arising from deep within your core, a glowing emanating light in your sacral chakra, at the base of your spine. As you inhale, picture flickers of golden, shimmering strands pouring in through the top of your head from an endless, eternal well. With each inhale, the golden strands become brighter and stronger, less like sunrays and more like shooting stars.

4. As you exhale, visualize these strands of light being carried on your breath and going into your partner's inhales, as their exhales become your inhales. You're giving and receiving them to each other in a never-ending cycle.

5. With each breath, you're more aware. More still. Try to keep your eyes open, but if it helps you to close them at first as you visualize, go ahead. And if your mind wanders or you find yourself giggling or becoming distracted, that's okay. Just come back to your breath and receive the moment and your experiences without judgment.

Do this exercise for five to ten minutes on a weekly basis, or anytime you need a connection recharge after a difficult argument or a period of time apart. And if you are single, try it by yourself as you gaze into your own eyes in the mirror. You can also use this exercise before sex or self-stimulation to heighten your pleasure and connection.

DEEPENING YOUR SEXUAL EXPERIENCE WITH TAOISM

Taoism (or Daoism) is a spiritual practice that originated in China over 3,500 years ago. Tao means the way of the universe and the qi or chi (the energy) of the universe. Taoists seek to balance their chi with the universe and live in harmony with all beings.

In Taoism, sex is seen as healing and restorative. It is referred to as HiQi, meaning "joining energy." Many Taoists believe that HiQi can lengthen your lifespan because the joining of your energy with another will revitalize and sustain both of you.

HiQi (and Taoism in general) is built on the idea that the universe is composed of yin and yang energy. Yang is the masculine energy that can be understood as similar to Shiva, and yin is the feminine energy that can be understood as similar to the Hindu goddess Shakti.

Yet while Tantra treats the body as a gateway to a higher consciousness, Taoism treats the body as home base. Taoism is focused on the health and caretaking of what is happening in the here and now, with our physical forms and senses. It complements Tantra perfectly, as it allows us to marry both the physical and spiritual in perfect harmony. Tantra gives us the wings, while Taoism gives us the gravity that allows us to balance and ground.

I find that bringing Taoist practices into sex can be incredibly beneficial for people who are feeling disconnected from their partner. Tantra can give us the healing and liberating aspects of sex, but Taoism can give us the connection and the security we need as well.

Many people wrongly view Taoism as a passive spiritual state, which doesn't align with the idea of a powerful and passionate sex life. But although "nonaction" is one of the principal ideas of Taoism, this doesn't mean inactivity or powerlessness. Instead, it means receptivity. When you practice Taoist ideas, you are open to whatever life may bring you, and you are prepared to meet and experience every sensation as it comes. Picture a flower as it receives everything from sunlight, to raindrops, to moonlight, to snowflakes. The flower doesn't resist or fight these experiences. But nor is it passive. It is still in integrity with its purpose, whether it is blooming or being pollinated or ending its life cycle.

Taoist Inner Smile Meditation

The following Taoist meditation is a wonderful way to shift into a higher vibration at any time, including as a prelude to sex. I also often recommend it as a regular practice to alleviate anxiety and stress and get us into a more playful and sexy mood. In the Taoist Inner Smile meditation, we quite literally "smile" into different parts of the body, sending positive energy there. It's quite simple and feels wonderful in mind and body!

1. Begin by grounding yourself as you now know how to do.
2. Create a source of smiling energy in your mind. You can imagine your own smiling face, or that of someone or something you love. Perhaps you just think back to a memory or time in which you felt deep peace. I often just imagine the shape of a smile in my mind. Just get a sense of the smile's energy, the feeling of it.
3. Once you have that sense of a smile, imagine the *energy* of that joyful smiling face or image there, three feet in front of you.
4. Place your awareness on the midpoint between your eyebrows, the area considered the "third eye." Let your forehead relax as

THE ANCIENT WISDOM OF TANTRA, KUNDALINI, AND TAOISM

you do so. Imagine drawing in this beautiful, smiling energy in front of you. Imagine that smiling energy accumulating at the mid-eyebrow. Let it overflow into your body.

5. Smile into your eyes. Feel the joyful energy shine into them.

6. Send the energy down to your neck, moving down to the collarbone. Your entire throat and shoulders are bathed in smiling light.

7. Smile into your chest, your heart, ribs, intestines, all your organs, your uterus (if you have one), your pelvis, your legs, arms, and all over your body. Smile into them in the same way that you just smiled into your eyes until every organ and every cell of your body that you can think of is bathing in the light of a loving smile.

Taoism in the Bedroom

Keep in mind that in the bedroom, Taoism encourages us to bring thoughtfulness into how we choose our partners. Taoists believe that subtle energies are exchanged during sex, so if you have sex with someone who doesn't align with your values, you could be taking on that energy. Taoists also don't believe in meaningless sex, because even though having sex raises your chi, it also releases chi. You will not be in balance with the universe if you are expanding your energy with several partners and have your attention and energies divided.

The energy exchange of sex is not to be taken lightly. Nor is the lack of energy exchange. That is why when people aren't having sex with their partner, they can feel so disconnected and loveless, even if they are still connecting in other ways that aren't physical. We need that flow of chi between us to keep us in harmony and to elevate us.

As part of this energy exchange, Taoists often practice what is known as yin pu yang for men and yang pu yin for women. This is the practice of having sexual relations without reaching orgasm. Yin pu yang means to gather a woman's yin for the purpose of enhancing the male yang, while yang pu yin means gathering a man's yang to enhance the female yin.

The ability to delay orgasm or deny orgasms entirely is not easy, and as such this practice of yin pu yang was taught in secret and learned over many years. But you don't have to become a Taoist scholar to apply this ancient wisdom to your own sexual experiences.

For those with penises, delaying orgasm or learning how to have a "retrograde" orgasm is an exciting way to level up your sex life *and* increase your chi. Research shows that the average orgasm lasts for about thirty seconds or less. But with retrograde ejaculation exercise, you can last as long as you want. This is how singer Sting achieves his reported twenty-four-hour orgasms! Not to mention, in the Tantric tradition, semen retention allows men to retain life force that energizes them in ways ejaculation can limit.

Retrograde ejaculation occurs when semen flows backward into the bladder instead of out of the urethra. In women, this can also happen; it is estimated that up to 50 percent of women will experience female ejaculation during intimacy at some point in their lives. But, as with men, instead of the ejaculate coming out of the urethra, it goes back into the woman's bladder.

Retrograde ejaculation essentially involves orgasm without ejaculation. This means that if, on an arousal scale of zero to ten (ten being ejaculation), you want to keep yourself from arriving at a ten (ejaculation), never reach that point, at least until your next sexual encounter.

Steps for Retrograde Ejaculation

This exercise provides instructions for people with penises. Learn to experience retrograde ejaculation and keep orgasmic feelings alive for hours instead of seconds!

1. When you are becoming aroused, pause before you reach the point of orgasm. (If orgasm is a ten, pause around a seven.)
2. Apply pressure to the area. You can do this by squeezing the base of the penis or by pressing the area between your perineum and scrotum or the perineum and anus. For the record, the perineum is the area between the scrotum and anus (or vagina and anus). By putting pressure here, you can "redirect" your ejaculate. The pressure shouldn't be painful; it should just feel very, very good. Try using the "finger lock" technique to make sure you are on the right spot. This is when you place the tips of your ring finger and middle finger on top of your index finger, then push downward to create firm steady pressure right on your perineum.
3. As you reach orgasm, visualize that energy moving back into your body rather than exploding outward. Visualize yourself as a sandy beach soaking up all that salty water and expanding with that energy and life-nurturing fluid.
4. You can make this exercise even more powerful by applying pressure at the base of your spine when you reach orgasm. This area is ripe with sexual energy and power. When you put pressure at the base of the spine, you can visualize your sexual energy traveling up your spine and exploding out the top of your head at your crown chakra.

Try this technique alone during self-stimulation and then play with this exercise while having sex with your partner. It's okay if you reach orgasm and ejaculate. This will be a learning curve, and all orgasms are good orgasms in my book!

One cautionary note here: retrograde ejaculation, or "dry ejaculation" means that by simultaneously squeezing the base of the penis or applying pressure to the perineum, the semen, instead of coming out the penis, goes back up the urethra into the bladder and is released from the body with the next urination. The risk with retrograde ejaculation is that it is considered a condition of infertility. So if you are a male seeking to impregnate someone, avoid retrograde as a regular practice.

Sexpiration Meditation

The sexpiration meditation is an exercise I created to help to experience and enhance the sexual energy moving through your body. This process is based on the concept of the microcosmic orbit. Also known as the small heavenly circulation, the microcosmic orbit is a fundamental practice in Taoist meditation and QiGong. It involves the conscious circulation of Qi (Chi), or life energy, through two primary energy channels in the body: the governing vessel, which runs up the spine, and the conception vessel, which runs down the front of the body. By focusing on and guiding the flow of Qi through these channels, practitioners aim to balance and harmonize their internal energy, enhance physical health, and deepen their spiritual awareness.

The key to this exercise is the pelvic bowl (the area between your hip bones, where your pelvic floor and internal sexual organs reside, connected to your external sexual organs). To work with the pelvic bowl, it helps to imagine a long, shallow, and beautiful bowl resting gently inside your pelvis, in the space between your hip bones. It can be made of any material that appeals to or inspires you: alabaster, crystal, or any material you would like.

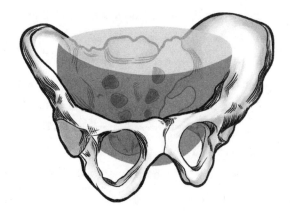

The pelvic bowl

The other important key to this exercise is the Kegel muscles. Your Kegels are the muscles that are shaped like a figure eight, encircling the vaginal opening or scrotum and the anus. These are the same muscles we use to stop the flow of urine midstream. (You'll learn a lot more about working with your Kegels in the coming chapters.) To listen to a guided version of this meditation, go to drlauraberman.com/sexmagic.

1. Take a few clearing breaths and ground yourself in your body.
2. Imagine a beautiful, bright light pouring in through the top of your head. As you breathe in deeply, the light pours into your body, filling every cell, every muscle, every corner and organ with light. This is a healing, beautiful, sparkling light. Notice the color of the light. As you inhale, visualize the light

flowing into your body. As you exhale, visualize the light spreading out like a wave from your head to your toes.

3. Put your attention on your heart chakra, the energy center in the center of your chest. (For more on chakras, see chapter 3.) As you breathe in the light, send it to your heart and let the light intensify. As you breathe out, the heart center is relaxing, opening, and expanding like a flower. As your heart expands and opens, you can send your light out to another person—someone you love, want to connect with, or want to heal. Maybe for now you just keep the light centered on your own heart.

4. Your body is filled with and flowing with light. It's time to put your awareness on the pelvic bowl. Now, as you breathe in, imagine the light flowing in through your head and down to your pelvis. The pelvic bowl lengthens out to receive it. As you breathe out, squeeze the Kegel muscles and imagine the bowl settling snugly into your pelvis, with light pooling in it, beginning to fill it. Do this for several breaths until you feel your pelvic bowl is filled with light.

5. Try looping the energy. Put your attention on that glittering pool of precious, oily light in your pelvic bowl. Imagine that your spine is like a straw. As you take small sipping breaths in (like you are sucking through a straw), squeeze the Kegels, propelling the light out of the bowl into and up your spine. Imagine the light is being sucked up the straw with your breath, all the way up the spine over the top of your head. As you breathe out slowly and smoothly, the light flows through your brow chakra, the energy center between your eyes, and down through the front of your body back into the pelvic bowl. Repeat this circle several times.

THE ANCIENT WISDOM OF TANTRA, KUNDALINI, AND TAOISM

Once you've practiced the sexpiration meditation on your own and feel like you've mastered the flow, be sure to try it during sex by yourself or with someone else. Use the meditation to pull and pool the sexual sensations that you feel building in your genitals into the pelvic bowl. Then use your intention, Kegels, and sipping breaths to intensify the arousal in the same way as in this exercise. Pull the energy up the straw of your spine and circle it through your body for full-body, erotic, energetic sensations!

Nine Thrusts Technique

The "Nine Thrusts Technique" is an ancient Taoist technique, the purpose of which is to create a pattern of thrusting that is deeply pleasurable for both partners. You can use this for vaginal penetration or anal penetration, or you can use dildos or other sex aids if you don't have a partner with a penis.

First, make sure you are in a position that allows for the partner with the penis (or the partner with the toy) to fully control the depth of penetration. It's also a great idea to have extra lubricant on hand.

The Nine Thrusts Technique combines more shallow thrusts (which are yang-oriented) and deeper, slower strokes (which are more yin). The sequence goes like this:

1. 9:1 Shallow to Deep: To start with, the partner who is penetrating inserts only the head of the penis or toy into the vagina (or anus). The partner does this nine times. Then, they insert the entire penis or toy in a deep thrust, just once.

2. 8:2 Shallow to Deep: Next, the penetrating partner uses eight shallow strokes followed by two deep strokes. They then go

on in this way, decreasing the number of shallow strokes by one and increasing the deep strokes by one.

3. 7:3 Shallow to Deep
4. 6:4 Shallow to Deep
5. 5:5 Shallow to Deep
6. 4:6 Shallow to Deep
7. 3:7 Shallow to Deep
8. 2:8 Shallow to Deep
9. 1:9 Shallow to Deep

That's a total of ninety strokes! While you can choose the pace, slower is definitely better. But varying the strokes does build sexual tension and intensify the experience. To add another level, the receiving partner can squeeze their Kegels, contracting them during the deep strokes or withdrawals. And remember, practice makes perfect, so don't worry if you lose count.

SEX MAGIC CASE FILE

"I'm a fighter," Bo said to me proudly during our first session.

He certainly was. Bo (short for Bogart) had a more storied life than almost anyone I had ever met. He survived a childhood with one incarcerated parent and another parent who was a severe alcoholic and cannabis addict. In fact, Bo had been named by his father, not for the famous 1950s movie actor Humphrey Bogart, but as a tongue-in-cheek nod to the colloquial stoner term for hogging the joint, "bogarting." As an adult, Bo also survived a motorcycle wreck, skin cancer, bankruptcy, and two divorces.

With his buzzed haircut and sleeves of tattoos, Bo looked every inch the "biker dude" he described himself to be. His green eyes

THE ANCIENT WISDOM OF TANTRA, KUNDALINI, AND TAOISM

shined with mirth and wit as he told me about his many adventures, including the time he almost got arrested at customs in Honduras.

Needless to say, Bo was a badass, and he wasn't afraid to let me know it.

But I knew there was vulnerability and fear behind the tougher aspects of his personality. I heard the quiver in his voice when he talked to me about his mom's arrest when Bo was just five years old, and I saw the tears in his eyes when he told me his wife was threatening to leave him.

"Meredith is my everything," said Bo. "She's the reason I was able to quit drinking and finally stay quit. She's the reason I was able to get stable enough to talk to my kids again. She's the only woman who has ever really *got* me. She's more than my soulmate, she's my soul, you know?"

I felt the warmth and light emanating from Bo as he described his wife of twelve years. But their love story wasn't perfect, far from it. Over the years, the couple had broken up and made up more times than I could track, and Bo's alcohol and drug use had made their relationship intense and painful. Even now that he was sober from all substances, Meredith still felt disconnected and unsafe in her relationship with Bo.

"I don't get it," says Bo. "I know I messed up a lot in our marriage, but I haven't touched a drink in over three years. I don't lash out and rage the way I used to. I'm gentler and kinder—she says so herself. But she says I'm a 'dry drunk,' and that she still can't connect with me . . . I have no idea what she's talking about! We're together 24-7 and I basically never stop talking."

We both laughed, but I already knew exactly what Meredith was talking about. Bo was energy in motion, completely frank and almost shockingly honest, but he also had a wary demeanor that made me feel like he was waiting for the other shoe to drop. Waiting for someone to abandon him. Waiting for someone to hurt him so he could say, "See, I knew you were going to do that, so I don't care, and you didn't hurt me."

Bo and Meredith also weren't having sex anymore. "I don't really enjoy sex since I stopped the booze," confessed Bo. "I still think she's damn sexy, but it's just hard for me to finish . . . I don't mind pleasing her and making her happy, but when she wants me to cum, I just get in my head too much. She gets offended and cries. It kills me, but I don't know why she just can't be happy with me being the giver. Most women would kill for that, wouldn't they?"

But Meredith didn't want just orgasms. She wanted authentic connection and living intimacy, an exchange between the two of them, not just a performance on Bo's part.

I knew that the part of Bo that was keeping him from being able to connect with his wife was deeply serving Bo in some way, otherwise he wouldn't have been so deeply entrenched with this part of himself. I just needed to help him find out who that part was, and how he could learn to love and care for this part without allowing it to dictate all of his other parts.

Over the course of several sessions, I learned so much about Bo and how his mind had adapted to protect himself in the face of great trauma. Not only did he witness his mother being arrested when he was a little boy (an incredibly traumatic experience for a child), but his mom later went on to be convicted and spent the majority of Bo's childhood behind bars. Bo was rarely able to visit because the prison was several hours away. Instead, he was raised by his father, who was often inebriated and unreliable.

Although Bo was adamant that his father was a "damn good single dad" and never abused him, the truth was that Bo spent a lot of

THE ANCIENT WISDOM OF TANTRA, KUNDALINI, AND TAOISM

time alone growing up. He was often neglected and left to fend for himself, making ketchup sandwiches for dinner while his dad was out with friends or getting wasted in their basement.

In addition, Bo grew up severely bullied. He was raised in the 1970s in a small town with a religious conservative community and bigoted beliefs about single parents and alcohol use. "We didn't have any other family, and the kids in town were really mean to me. They threw rocks at me when I walked by. I never really understood why I was rejected by them, I just knew I was bad. I figured finding a girl, getting married, and having kids would give me someone to count on and help me fit in. I thought I would feel normal, but instead I still just felt like a fraud. I love my kids but I was so depressed and anxious all the time when they were growing up."

"Because you inherently felt the real you wasn't enough. Nothing and no one in your life had told you otherwise," I observed.

"Yep," sighed Bo. "But I could never admit that. So instead I drank too much and cheated on my wife. Then another, then another."

Finally, at thirty-seven years old, Bo stopped running and got sober.

"I know I will never drink or do drugs again," says Bo. "Meredith believes me when I say that. I have proven my commitment to sobriety. But she says I still haven't proven my commitment to her. I don't know how she can say that. I literally picked her and our life together over the medicine that had been keeping me going most of my life."

"But she still feels like you don't love her enough to let her in," I said, harkening back to an earlier comment Bo had shared with me. "But I think it's not that you don't love her enough; I think it's that you're scared of the damage she could do if she leaves you."

"No, not just that," said Bo. "I'm not just afraid of the damage she could cause. I am afraid of the damage she could *find*."

With this one statement, we discovered Bo's core wound and the part of himself that was blocking him from truly loving and being able to be truly loved in return. He was not just terrified of being left; he had the core belief that he deserved to be left. As a child, he didn't know how to process his mother's incarceration and his dad's drinking and disappearing acts. Kids have egocentric minds, meaning that they think everything that happens in their world is related to them or because of them. So, in a way, Bo felt deeply responsible that he wasn't "good enough" to have a stable home and "normal" parents like the other kids in his community.

All of this amounted to making Bo not only afraid of trusting people and being hurt again but being "found out" by the people he most wanted to love him. It was as though he needed to hide his "badness," so he constructed elaborate walls around himself, including in the bedroom. Without the assistance of alcohol, Bo couldn't allow himself to be vulnerable to be pleasured and to reach orgasm with his wife. It was almost as though he didn't believe he deserved to be adored and loved in this way.

Once we were able to start meeting and healing these parts of Bo, he was able to grow into creating the sex life he had been wishing for his entire adult life. As part of this process, I knew he needed to unblock his root chakra and build a sense of security within himself. Bo and I spent the next three months working together on processing some of his trauma, shifting his limiting beliefs, and cultivating, opening, and supporting his root chakra. He tried yoga for the first time and loved it, regularly practicing poses that made him feel grounded and safe in his body. He spent a lot of time in nature and discovered that he found tremendous healing with the grounding practice I taught him. He got clearer and clearer on what he needed to feel safe to be open and vulnerable with Meredith, and the two of them came for several couples' sessions together.

Feeling deeply supported by the Earth and held by the universe's expansive and eternal embrace was the key in helping Bo to fall into pure pleasure.

It took several months, but we slowly found ways for Bo to start letting pleasure in. Meredith gave him sensual massages, and they went skinny dipping at a hot spring near their favorite hiking trail. They rebuilt their intimacy from the inside out, because despite the fact that they had been together for years, they had both learned to hide their vulnerabilities and needs from each other. The result was not only the passionate and connective sex life that they both needed, but also a more joyful life for Bo overall.

"I used to think sobriety just meant not drinking and not doing drugs," he said. "But I have found sobriety means so much more than that. It means actively choosing connection over isolation. It means reaching out instead of lashing out; it means asking for help instead of hiding."

It means, in other words, seeking out the barriers we have built between us and love, and greeting those barriers with tender curiosity and gentle hands. And soon we find that those barriers become portals, secret passageways that are here to bring us to the next level of consciousness and connection.

CHAPTER 3

A Sex Magician's Guide to the Chakra System

Your body is the harp of your soul, and it is yours to bring forth sweet music from it or confused sounds.

—Kahlil Gibran

Everything, from the tiniest blade of grass to the highest mountain, is radiating energy. Each cell in our bodies emits energy in different ways, depending on its location in the body and its job. We touched on the chakras in the previous chapter, but now it's time to take a deeper dive into this powerful system of energy centers running through the human body. Originating from ancient Hindu and Buddhist spiritual traditions, *chakra* is a Sanskrit word that that translates to "wheel." However, the chakras are actually more like energy vortexes than wheels. They serve to work with and distribute energy between your body and the world around you. The chakras spin in a clockwise direction when moving energy out of your body into the field around you, and they spin counterclockwise when pulling energy into your body from the world (and people) around you.

The seven main chakras are located at specific points along the spine, from its base to the crown of the head: root (Muladhara), sacral (Svadhisthana), solar plexus (Manipura), heart (Anahata), throat (Vishuddha), third eye (Ajna), and crown (Sahasrara) chakras. These are the energy centers that directly impact different areas of the body and spirit. Chakras need to be open and flowing to serve us most effectively. If your chakras are closed or inactive—or alternately *over*active—you will notice this throughout your life, including your sex life.

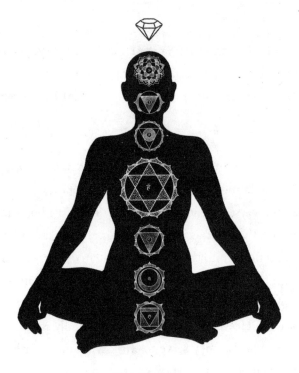

The Chakras

We can further understand the energy of our chakras by understanding the color associated with each of them. Visible light emits electromagnetic waves that oscillate through the field across time and space. The speed of these oscillations determines the color our eyes perceive. For example, red light has a lower frequency and appears as a gentle wave, while purple light has a higher frequency, with rapid peaks and troughs. These waves can be measured in nanometers, allowing us to determine their energy levels.

Although each of the chakras has a very distinct and different role in our bodies and our souls, they *all* influence us as sexual beings. Following is a quick rundown of the chakras. If you'd like to take a more extensive dive into the subject, you can check out my book *You're Not Crazy, You're Just Ascending.*

THE ROOT (MULADHARA) CHAKRA

This chakra, located in the tailbone area, is associated with the color red. This chakra *roots* us and gives us grounding and stability. It's the seat of safety in ourselves, with others, and with the universe.

Our root chakra gives us the base we need for raw, authentic sexual experiences. But when it's blocked, it can cause sexual pain and even prevent us from reaching orgasm. Our root chakra is associated with our fight-flight-freeze-or-fawn reflex. The freeze reflex and the fawn reflex have recently been added to our understanding of how these primal adrenaline-fueled behaviors appear differently in men and women. The freeze reflex is just as it sounds, like that of a deer frozen in headlights or a bunny freezing in the grass when it hears a twig snap. The fawn reflex happens when someone who is in danger reverts to "fawning," pretending to be enthused and happy as they plot and wait for their escape from the dangerous situation. This recent addition came about as we've begun to better understand how primal reactions appear differently in men and women.

If you experienced trauma in your life, especially sexual trauma, your root chakra is likely imbalanced. But you might not even realize that you're in a fawning state or a freeze state during sex if you don't know what you desire or need in a sexual exchange. If you find yourself lying inactive during sex and waiting for your partner to *do* things to you while your mind is a million miles away, this is certainly a blocked root chakra. On other hand, if you're more focused on performing like you're in a porn movie with excessive moaning that isn't authentic, you might be locked in a fawn reflex. Trying to hyper-please your partner and being afraid to express any sexual needs or refusing any sexual favor are signs that your root chakra could be overactivated.

THE SACRAL (SVADHISTHANA) CHAKRA

The sacral chakra is associated with the color orange, and it is connected to pleasure, creativity, sexuality, and fertility. Our sacral chakra is very important to our sex life. It is the seat of our sexuality, and it governs our sexual energy. This includes our libido, our sexual response, and our sexual self-worth. An overactive sacral chakra will present as someone who can't control their emotions and is always swinging from one extreme to the next, especially as it relates to their romantic relationships. One moment they're convinced their partner is the best thing since sliced bread; the next minute they're threatening them with divorce. In the bedroom, an overactive sacral chakra will look like someone who is ruled by their sexual desires. They might struggle with watching too much porn or flirting excessively and seeking sexual attention in order to feel important and valued.

An underactive sacral chakra could present as someone who struggles to feel sexual desire. They might not have sexual fantasies, or any fantasies: Creativity is also a key role of the sacral chakra, so

A SEX MAGICIAN'S GUIDE TO THE CHAKRA SYSTEM

when your sacral chakra is blocked, you might feel like you have no imagination or ingenuity.

THE SOLAR PLEXUS (MANIPURA) CHAKRA

This chakra is located right below your ribs in the center of your chest and is represented by the color yellow. It's the center of our worth and boundaries with how we want to be treated.

The solar plexus chakra is the throne of our personal power. If your solar plexus chakra is underactive, you will struggle with expressing your personal truth and standing in your own power. You will be easily influenced by others, and easily impacted by others. You will struggle with willpower and sticking to what you believe is important, which only makes you feel more powerless.

Someone with an overactive solar plexus will always want to be in charge or will feel afraid to express vulnerability, and their sex life will suffer as a result. If you're a man, this might look like intense fear of emasculation. You might refuse to go to therapy with your partner. You may not have authentic conversations about your inner world. If you're a woman, this might look like a fear of trusting or depending on a man. I often find that women with an overactive solar plexus will be incredibly ambitious and successful. They are often super moms who do it all, but then wind up feeling resentful that their partner never pitches in, even as they criticize and micromanage when their partner does try to get involved. It's easy to see how this dynamic can poison a couple's sex life. She won't feel sexy because she feels like his mom, and she doesn't feel as attracted to her partner because she has taken away their power—meanwhile the partner's desire suffers too because they now feel like a scolded child rather than a desirable and powerful lover.

THE HEART (ANAHATA) CHAKRA

This chakra sits in the middle of our chests. Associated with the color green, it represents pure love and compassion, for others and for ourselves. The heart chakra is also believed to hold the "pilot light" of our soul, meaning it houses the tiny eternal flame that is and was the beginning of our life here.

The heart chakra is our source of unconditional love and compassion. Many people say that they can feel the heart chakra instantly activated when they see their children or snuggle their pets. But your heart chakra also has an important role in intimacy and is very influential in your sex life. If your heart chakra is blocked, you will struggle to connect with your emotional side during sex. You won't be able to feel the depth that you crave during sex, and your partner will likely feel this disconnect as well.

An overactive heart chakra will look like someone who *pours* out intimacy. They struggle with codependency and feeling their own feelings. In the bedroom, someone with an overactive heart chakra might struggle to feel present and in their body because they're so hyper-focused on how their partner is feeling and what they might be thinking. They are very sensitive to any possible sign that their partner isn't happy with them, and they might battle jealousy and insecurity, always fearing that they'll be cheated on or abandoned for not being satisfying or good enough.

Access Your Heart's Eternal Flame

Spiritually speaking, the heart's eternal flame is a representation of the infinite and unending source of love, compassion, and divine connection within each of us. This flame is often seen as the core of one's being, the initial pilot light of our consciousness. It's the spark of our soul, embodying the purest form of spiritual energy that fuels our capacity for kindness, empathy, and emotional warmth. Nurturing this eternal heart flame opens the heart chakra and centers us in loving energy. It's a beautiful way to stay connected to love and to infuse deep, loving energy into any sexual encounter. If you'd like to cultivate a connection to your own heart's flame, here's how.

1. Sit or lie down comfortably, close your eyes, and ground, as you learned to do in chapter 1.
2. Now, do a body scan. Imagine you are scanning your entire body starting at the top of the head and slowly traveling all the way down to your feet. Imagine your awareness like a light that is gently scanning down your whole body, noticing places of tightness or density. You don't have to do anything with this information. Just register the sensations, because this is your baseline to see how you feel after this exercise.
3. Put your conscious awareness in the center of your chest, right where the heart chakra resides. Visualize a small but powerful flame in the center of your heart chakra. This is the spark that is your beginning, the core of your consciousness and one of the key points of your divine connection. It's like a pilot light. If you are a spiritual person, this flame could be God's love for you and your eternal connection to that unconditional love. But this flame could also represent your connection to nature, to your Source, to Mother Earth, to the love that flows through you and all around you. Your flame will be different from anyone else's flame, but in the end it will feel instantly recognizable to you. When you've reached that flame, you will know it.

4. If you're struggling to get there, try thinking of your most precious memory. Maybe it was lying on the beach by your partner on a romantic vacation. Maybe it is when you see your beloved dog's face. Think of a time when you felt imbued by love and buoyed by love, utterly lifted, and filled with that indestructible pure light. Let that be the flame.

5. Now, lean into that flame. Let it get brighter and stronger. Imagine it getting so big that it fills your whole body. Feel it warming you from the tips of your toes to the ends of your hair. Bask there for at least five minutes—the longer the better!

6. Try imagining the heart's flame spreading even wider, beyond the edges of your body and into the room around you, even out into the world or to others to whom you want to spread love. How does it feel when you are connected to your Source?

7. Now, do another body scan. From this state of unconditional love, what physical feelings do you notice? Is your chest more open, your muscles looser, tingling, or warm? Do you notice a difference in the density or tightness you felt at the beginning of this exercise?

THE THROAT (VISHUDDHA) CHAKRA

This chakra is right where you think it would be, in your throat. It is connected to the color blue and is associated with communication, but specifically the ability to communicate your truth and express your true authentic self.

The throat chakra is the home of communication and expression, but not just any self-expression. This isn't the chakra for small talk or surface-level intimacy. Instead, this is the chakra that rules how much of ourselves we communicate with others. If you have been unable to express your gender identity or sexual orientation, this can lead to a blocked throat chakra. If you haven't been able to express your sexual fantasies or your sexual desire, such as if you grew up in a very conservative and religious home, your throat chakra might be blocked.

So what does an overactive throat chakra look like? Someone who is afraid of silence and stillness. Someone who needs constant reassurance and compliments from their partner in the bedroom, or who constantly seeks validation from the opposite sex when it comes to how they look and how sexually desirable they are. Someone whose throat chakra is overactive might not be able to stop oversharing, even to the detriment of their relationship. For example, they might tell friends or family about their personal sex life or intimacy, even when their partner asks them to keep it private. They might not take care with how they share their sexual—or other—needs, accidentally creating careless communications or hurt feelings.

THE THIRD EYE (AJNA) CHAKRA

In between our brows, the third eye is the chakra that can intuit and imagine, and it's associated with the color indigo. It is our connection to the unseen and the unknowable. It is our ability to see and know things that are beyond what reality may show us.

The third eye chakra governs our ability to see the unseen. It is the gateway through which we can access our intuition and our deepest wisdom. If you want to elevate your sexual experiences, a blocked third eye chakra can prevent this. If you feel stuck or can't figure out the correct path in life or are always questioning your purpose, you might have a blocked third eye chakra. In the bedroom, this might mean you feel a disconnect or a lack of spiritual energy between your partner and you. You might feel like you are cut off from sexual meaning or from connecting with your partner as deeply as you want to.

An overactive third eye chakra will appear like someone who isn't grounded. They have their head in the clouds and aren't proactive about following through on real-life goals and plans. They might have lots of lofty ideas about how they want to improve their sex life or their relationship, but they get lost in the weeds when it comes to putting their plans into action. They also might be very distracted or even dissociated during sex, not necessarily due to trauma but to being too focused on the spirit realms and not present in the body.

THE CROWN (SAHASRARA) CHAKRA

The crown chakra is located on the top of the head. Represented by purple, this chakra is our knowing chakra. This is where we access divine energy, and get "downloads" or messages from the spirit realm. This chakra holds our wisdom and our awareness, what we know and all that's possible to know.

The crown chakra is our connection to the spiritual world. We need a balanced crown chakra to experience the sacred side of sex. If your crown chakra is underactive, you're going to approach sex without gravity or importance. You won't take sexual activity as sacredly as you'd like to, whereas if your crown chakra is overactive, you might struggle to loosen up and enjoy the silliness and joy of the physical aspects of sex.

When the crown chakra is activated and open during sex, intimacy becomes divinely inspired. The crown chakra is also the access point for having, quite literally, mind-blowing orgasms.

DON'T FORGET THE POWER OF THE DIAMOND CHAKRA

While most refer only to seven chakras, there is an eighth chakra known as the diamond chakra. It is our portal chakra, the one that connects us to other dimensions and other divine beings, including those who have gone on before us and those we have yet to know.

This chakra is our connection not only to the spiritual world, but also to and through our most essential selves: to our past lives and our future lives and to our soul's purpose here and now. When you are connected to this chakra during sex, you will have the ability to have truly transformative sex that will feel unlike anything you have ever experienced before. You will feel like your intimacy is being divinely supported, and sacred.

I love connecting to my diamond chakra when I need to feel spiritual support or want to ask for spiritual guidance. And when you tap into your diamond chakra before or during sex, it makes sex a seriously spiritual experience, not to mention that you will receive divine messages in the high-frequency sexual state.

Tap In and Tune In to Your Diamond Chakra

1. Close your eyes and take some deep breaths. Ground yourself.
2. Put all of your conscious awareness on the bottom tip of the diamond chakra above your head. Picture it like the tip at the bottom of a perfectly faceted diamond. It's a tiny pinprick of light right there about twelve inches above your head.
3. Gently hold your attention there on that point. As you hold this gentle focus, you will feel a subtle pull upward or a sensation of plugging in. I always know when I am plugged into my diamond chakra because my ears pop. But if you don't feel

anything, don't worry. As you practice and keep your attention there, you will likely experience a similar physical sign that you are on the right path. And even if you don't feel it, the connection is always there.

4. Once you feel yourself plugged in, call in your guides and higher self by saying or thinking, "I am calling in my guides, only those aligned with the highest frequency and for my highest good, to deliver divinely inspired messages to me in this high-frequency sexual state."

5. Now you can begin self-stimulation or even a sexual encounter. If you hold quiet, openhearted curiosity, you will receive beautiful information or the answer to a question.

HOW TO BALANCE AND OPEN YOUR CHAKRAS

I could write an entire book on the nuances of healing, opening, and balancing the chakras, and there are many experts who have done so. If you'd like to take a deeper dive, I get into it in great detail in my books *Quantum Love* and *You're Not Crazy, You're Just Ascending*, but here are some practical strategies that help heal all the chakras.

* **Cultivate the colors.** Wearing the color of the chakra you want to support is believed to help. For instance, if you struggle with a sense of groundedness and safety, wear red often, even just on your feet. Add a lot of green to your wardrobe if you want to open your heart chakra and connect more deeply to it.

* **Practice meditation and visualization.** Where attention goes, energy flows, as does healing. Any kind of meditation or mindfulness practice supports your mind and body and

A SEX MAGICIAN'S GUIDE TO THE CHAKRA SYSTEM

can be helpful in unblocking your chakras. During meditation, visualize the chakra you want to work on and see it as a pulsing, vibrant ball of energy. As you breathe in, the chakra fills with light. As you breathe out, the light intensifies.

* **Engage in chakra-supporting movement.** Activities like yoga, qigong, and tai chi are wonderful ways to cultivate calm and clarity, but also to activate, balance, and open your chakras.

* **Try acupuncture and Reiki.** While acupuncture and Reiki are very different, both are facilitated by a practitioner, such as of Chinese medicine, energy healer, Reiki Master, or holistic healer. They can help you to open and heal any struggling or blocked energy centers in the body.

* **Take inspired action.** If you feel that one or more of your chakras are blocked, there are infinite actions you can take every day to support them. Ideas will come to you, just from reading the descriptions of the chakras above. For instance, if your throat is blocked, your job is to begin speaking your truth as much as possible. If this concerns you, start with strangers and then move on to friends and family. If your heart chakra is blocked, consider the ways you might be willing to show more vulnerability or willingness to receive. If you'd like to cultivate your third eye, crown, or diamond chakras, spend more time in meditation and spiritual pursuits.

* **Spend time in nature.** Few places are as healing and supportive for our bodies' energy systems as being in nature. Mother Nature holds and maintains a perfect healing frequency. She never matches our energy, but when we spend time in nature, we match hers. In addition, when we walk barefoot on the earth or grass, we automatically ground our energy systems.

TAKE THE CHAKRA ELEVATOR TO FULL-BODY ORGASM

Are you ready to work with your chakras to begin to pull genital sensations up and have the experience of full-body orgasms? The Chakra Elevator is one of the best ways to do so. In this exercise, you are going to use the chakras you've just learned about to move sensual and sexual sensations up and through your entire system. This is an unbelievably powerful exercise that is best learned in stages.

This exercise also requires use of your Kegel muscles. You'll be learning a lot more about the Kegels and how to strengthen them in the next chapter. For now, it's just important to know that these are muscles that surround the anus and vagina or scrotum in a figure eight pattern. They are the same muscles you use to hold in or stop the flow of urine. During this exercise you will be squeezing and releasing them to help move the energy through your body.

A Note on Moving Sexual Energy Through the Body

Learning how to master and move sexual energy around your body can be challenging. I find it helps to envision sexual energy as a light-filled, sparkling oil. It's an image borrowed from the popular Ayurvedic treatment called Shirodhara, or third eye therapy. If you've ever had this treatment, you probably experienced its trancelike effects as the warm, wonderful-smelling oil is poured in a constant gentle stream onto your forehead.

Take the image of Shirodhara and see your body's energy as warm, beautiful, sparkling, light-filled oil that moves through you the way you direct and between you and your partner. In fact, Chinese medicine promotes the idea that where your attention goes your chi, or

How to Ride the Chakra Elevator

Start with the sensation that is in your genitals. This technique creates big and beautiful full body arousal (and orgasm), but can be a little complex to master at first without a little practice. It helps to start with self-stimulation, either with your hand or a device. Later you can do this while having sexual contact with a partner for (literally) mind-blowing arousal!

1. As you are engaging in sexual stimulation and arousal is happening, observe the sensations that are centered around the genitals or your root chakra. You may feel tingling or warmth there. Notice it. Take deep breaths in and out. As you breathe in, open your Kegels as wide as you can. As you breathe out, squeeze or tighten them. Does it intensify when you breathe in? How does the sensation differ as you breathe out?

2. Let the sexual sensations intensify. On the next in-breath, open your Kegels wide and envision pulling the sexual sensation up from the root chakra (your genitals) to the sacral chakra, which is just below the belly button. Then, as you breathe out, gently rest your Kegels and let the sensations drop back down to the root chakra. Practice this looping several times: pull the energy up from the root to the sacral chakra and, as you breathe out, let it drop back down.

3. Next, as you breathe in and open your Kegels, pulling the energy up to the sacral from the root, breathe out, tighten

your Kegels, and keep the sensation in the sacral chakra without dropping it back down to the root. Keep it circling and intensifying as you breathe, without dropping it back down to the root. Do this several times.

4. Once comfortable with that, pull the energy up with your next in-breath. Keep your Kegels open from the sacral chakra to the solar plexus, above your belly button, and below your heart. As you breathe out, let it drop down to the sacral chakra again. Do this several times. Then on the next out-breath, tighten your Kegels and keep the energy circling in your solar plexus, letting it intensify. As you breathe in, the energy intensifies. As you breathe out, tightening your Kegels, it pulsates.

5. Move on to pull energy from your solar plexus chakra to your heart chakra in the center of your chest in the same way as above. First, breathe in with open Kegels. Now pull the energy up and let it drop on the out-breath. Then after another in-breath, practice tightening the Kegels on the out-breath and keeping the energy circling in the heart.

6. From here, move the energy from the heart chakra to the throat in the same way, eventually holding it and circling it there. Then move on from the throat chakra to the third eye chakra between your eyebrows, and finally from the third eye to the crown chakra at the top of the head in the same way.

7. And finally, if you wish, blow the sensation out the top of the crown chakra. You can send it to the stars, or if you want to experience a powerful energy boost, let it flow back down around you like a waterfall.

A SEX MAGICIAN'S GUIDE TO THE CHAKRA SYSTEM

FIREBREATH FOR RELEASING AND MOVING SEXUAL ENERGY

Ready to take your chakra system a little further? Firebreath meditations are chakra-oriented orgasmic meditations that allow you to circle sexual sensations around your entire body and fuel and prime the chakras while you do so.

The goal is to breathe into each of your chakras, and while doing so, imagine the color of that chakra filling with its light. Then you begin circling the energy between the chakras, in smaller circles between two adjacent chakras and larger circles between two non-adjacent chakras. It's not complicated but it takes practice. Once you've mastered the circling breaths, it's extremely powerful to use this technique first during self-stimulation then during sex with a partner. The sexual stimulation you feel in your genitals, where the root chakra resides, will be pulled through your entire body, circling between and energizing the chakras and massively enhancing sensation throughout your entire body.

Of the two forms of the Firebreath meditation I will be sharing with you, Complex Firebreath is the more complicated one, as the name implies. However, as you move this powerful and beautiful energy up your body in circles, it will feel like it has taken on a life of its own by the time it reaches your upper chakras. Many tangibly feel the intensity rise as the energy moves upward.

Complex Firebreath

Here's how to practice the Complex Firebreath exercise:

SEX MAGIC

1. Lie on your back with your knees up and feet flat on the bed or other surface on which you are resting. Relax your jaw as you breathe in gently through your nose and exhale through your mouth.

2. Begin to rock your pelvis gently as you breathe in deeply, imagining that your breath is filling up your belly like a balloon as your back gently arches off the surface. When you breathe out, flatten your lower back.

3. Begin to squeeze your Kegels as you exhale.

4. As you breathe in, imagine energy pooling in your root chakra at the base of your spine. As you breathe out imagine the intensity and frequency of that energy building. You can also place a hand on the root chakra to help focus energy there.

5. Next, as you inhale, imagine pulling energy upward, starting from your root chakra into your sacral chakra, lighting it up with brilliant energy. As you exhale, imagine and feel the energy circling back down to the root chakra. Continue to move your energy between your root and sacral chakras in a circle, breathing in and feeling the energy rise, breathing out and letting it gently circle back down to the root. Repeat this circle several times. Usually, it will begin to feel like the energy is moving more easily, almost on its own. Continue to squeeze the Kegels as you exhale.

6. Next, make the circle wider, pulling the energy from your root chakra up to your solar plexus chakra. Keep rocking with the breath, gently arching the back with the inhale, then flattening the back and squeezing the Kegels with the exhale. Repeat several times, creating a circle between the root and solar plexus chakras.

A SEX MAGICIAN'S GUIDE TO THE CHAKRA SYSTEM

7. As you continue breathing and squeezing your Kegels, let the energy drop from your solar plexus to your sacral chakra and pull the energy up from your sacral chakra to your solar plexus, circling it there in the same way for several breaths.

8. Next, pull the energy up from your solar plexus to your throat chakra. Make some sounds if you aren't already. Perhaps you can sigh, moan, or vocalize some "ahs." This can feel liberating and help move energy. The energy may start moving in circles on its own as the momentum builds.

9. When ready, let the energy drop back to the heart chakra and breathe in, moving the energy up to your throat chakra, circling it there several times.

10. Next, start circling the energy between your throat and crown, followed by circling between your third eye and throat chakras. When you're sending energy to your third eye, try rolling your closed eyes up as if you are looking toward the top of your head. This will help your energy rise.

11. The next step is to begin to circle the energy between the throat chakra and the crown, followed by a smaller circle between the third eye and crown chakra.

12. Continue taking deep slow breaths and moving your hips as you circle the energy through your body.

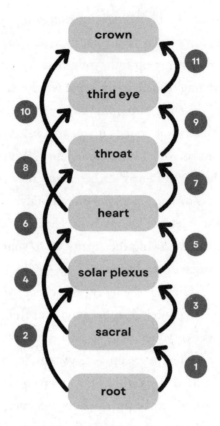

Complex Firebreath

Simple Firebreath

There is also a simpler version of the Firebreath exercise, where you just move up the chakras in order. Follow Complex Firebreath steps 1 through 6, but then simply move between two chakras at a time: root to sacral, sacral to solar plexus, solar plexus to heart, heart to throat, throat to third eye, and third eye to crown chakra. Keep breathing and moving your hips as the energy circles.

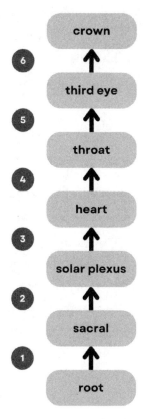

Simple Firebreath

SEX MAGIC CASE FILE

When your solar plexus is overactive, you might look like you have everything under control. You might even look like the most powerful person in the room.

That was Mercedes. She was a boss in more ways than one. Not only did she own her own Mexican restaurant and grocery store, she also was the matriarch of her huge, loving family, the queen of her many siblings, cousins, and relatives, many of whom worked at her store. Whether at work or at home, she was in charge and everyone knew it.

"I'm the oldest of seven kids," she confided in me when I apologized for running a few minutes late to our first session. "I am used to being patient."

I was intrigued by this revelation and asked her to tell me more about her childhood.

Mercedes explained that her parents immigrated to Texas from El Salvador when she was just two years old. By that time, they already had one-year-old twin boys, and Mercedes and four more siblings followed quickly over the years.

Mercedes's parents had to work hard to support their big family. Her dad was a migrant farmer who was often away for months at a time, meaning Mercedes was in charge of watching the younger kids while her mother worked double shifts as a waitress and as a nanny.

"She spent her days watching other people's kids, and I spent my days watching her kids," laughed Mercedes. "I was basically the mama. I did almost all of the cooking and cleaning. I was the one who took the kids to school and the dentist and the market."

"What about the twins? Were they any help to you? You were quite close in age," I noted.

Mercedes scoffed gently. "No, we were a typical Latino family," she said. "The men don't do much in the home. They never went to the laundromat once in their lives. Of course, they both had after-school jobs when they got old enough—before they got into a bad crowd, that is."

I felt a strong connection to Mercedes as she described her childhood. While my childhood experiences were very different from hers, I could relate to her experience of *parentification*—when a child takes on the role of a parent in the household. Mercedes certainly did that,

A SEX MAGICIAN'S GUIDE TO THE CHAKRA SYSTEM

acting as the physical and emotional stand-in for her mother since she couldn't be there herself.

"So you're used to being in charge," I said.

"Oh, *sí*, even now," says Mercedes. "I am the first person my siblings call when they need help. And as my parents get older and need more help, I feel like I am needed more than ever. I am the glue that holds everyone together. My restaurant keeps most of them employed. I don't know how my brothers would hold a job somewhere else, as lazy as they can be."

Her tone was sarcastic and a bit harsh. This was Mercedes's typical manner of speaking, and it was part of the reason she was in my office in the first place. Frank, her husband of thirteen years, was asking for a divorce. In my own sessions with Frank, he cited Mercedes's rage and her "attitude problem" as the main reasons.

"I promised I would get therapy," she said. "I promised I would do anything. He's giving me a chance . . . but I can tell it's just for show so he can prove to his parents and my parents that we tried."

Here, Mercedes started sobbing. It was the first show of emotion that she had displayed in the last hour. But after a few short sobs she quickly, almost angrily, wiped away the tears. I could sense how irritated she was with her tears, how she rejected her vulnerability with a visceral disgust.

I knew from my one-on-one session with her husband, Frank, that Mercedes didn't like to show emotions, except for anger.

"She's always sarcastic and lashing out at me," said Frank. "I feel like I am her emotional punching bag when things go wrong. If we are five minutes late somewhere or I forget something, she reacts like I just killed someone. I love her but I can't take it anymore. I kept thinking it would get better when the kids got older, but it's only gotten worse. I don't want to model this kind of relationship for my sons and daughters. They shouldn't think it's okay to talk to your partner in a nasty way just because you're irritated or something is going wrong."

Over my following sessions with Mercedes, we gently worked our way deeper into that anger, which she admitted was very real and often overwhelming. I could sense the anger locked in her body, in the way she held her posture and in the short, clipped way she spoke. Even when she was smiling, her eyes were tight and her body was taut with tension.

We began drawing that anger into the room with us, letting it out of the deep, dark recesses of Mercedes's heart, where it had been living for decades.

She hated to admit it, because it felt like a betrayal, but Mercedes was deeply resentful of her family. She was resentful that she didn't have a childhood because she was so busy caring for her parents' kids. She was resentful that her brothers got to run free while she was stuck at home changing diapers and washing bottles instead of enjoying her teenage years.

She was resentful that she was still her family's rock, still the one who took her mother to the doctor and helped bail her younger brothers out of trouble. Between her own kids and running her own business, Mercedes never did anything but care for others' needs.

On the one hand, this made her feel powerful and important. She was suited to being a leader, and she was very good at it. She liked being in charge and feeling like she had power. On the other hand, she was exhausted beyond measure. That exhaustion came out when she was at home with Frank, when she would blow a fuse over his tiny mistakes or forgetfulness.

When I asked Mercedes where in her body she felt her anger, she pointed to her chest.

A SEX MAGICIAN'S GUIDE TO THE CHAKRA SYSTEM

"It lives here," she said. "When I finally lay down at night, it feels like there is something sitting on top of me, suffocating me. It's hard to take a breath sometimes."

Mercedes also complained of mid-back pain, which made perfect sense. The solar plexus chakra is located in the center of our chest. But it is not just in the front of our bodies; so often when we have issues with our solar plexus chakra being over- or under-activated, symptoms will present both in our chest and in our back.

Mercedes also suffered from chronic digestive issues, including a lifelong struggle with ulcers and acid reflux. She blamed her diet, but despite lifestyle changes, her symptoms didn't abate.

I thought there might be other causes behind both her physical symptoms and her emotional symptoms. A blocked solar plexus chakra could be behind her flashes of rage, her extreme stubbornness, and her desire for control. It could also be causing her health issues.

At first Mercedes was somewhat resistant to chakra work. A devout Catholic, she was hesitant to consider new spiritual ideas. But she was desperate to save her marriage, and more important, her gut instinct was telling her to listen to me.

"I never heard the term 'solar plexus' before, but somehow what you're saying feels true. I trust you," she said, giving me a great compliment.

But she was still resistant to the idea that she had an anger problem.

"I know I have a temper, but I only lose it after people push me," she said. "If Frank would do what I asked or helped out more, I wouldn't get so angry at him. If my kids would do what they're told the first time, instead of making me ask a zillion times, I wouldn't have to scream at them."

We started to explore the first time she remembered feeling tightness in her chest and digestive issues. She recounted being so stressed at school that she would throw up and have to leave early, starting as early as sixth grade.

"My doctor said it could be hormones," she said. "But it always felt stress-related to me. There was just so much to do on school mornings. Getting all the kids breakfast and packing their lunches and getting them out to the bus on time. If they missed the bus, I had to take them on the train. Some days I felt like I was going to explode."

In other words, her solar plexus chakra had been heavily activated starting in childhood. She was essentially a twelve-year-old single mother, taking care of six siblings on her own, while still being a child herself. Her solar plexus chakra served her in many ways. It allowed her to be in control and to exert great power over younger siblings, ensuring they listened to her and stayed out of trouble.

But because there was never a moment when Mercedes got to be a child or take a break, her solar plexus chakra never got a chance to become balanced. She became rigid and highly critical, quick to push people around to get her way, and quick to lash out when people made what she viewed as silly mistakes.

I felt that balancing Mercedes's solar plexus chakra and releasing those decades of buried energy would help to free her from some of the chronic issues that had plagued her adulthood and her romantic relationships.

First, I taught her *kaphalabhati*, also known as skull-shining breath. This powerful breathing technique is simple to do: Sit in a cross-legged position on the floor. Press your forefinger and thumb together on each hand. Take a deep, slow breath in through your nose then release the breath through the mouth with a forceful sharp exhale. Repeat. Each time you inhale, picture yourself building rich, yellow light in the center of your chest, and each time you exhale, you are pressing the light out of yourself with full intention. Feel the pressure in your chest get lighter with each exhale.

Next, I asked Mercedes to create a personal power altar in her office and in her bedroom. She was surprised by this request.

"I thought you wanted me to be softer, not harder," she laughed. "Shouldn't I be making an altar about being weaker, not stronger?"

I smiled.

"I don't want you to feel less powerful; I want you to feel *more* powerful," I said. "My theory is that a lot of your rage stems from the fact that you feel like things are out of your control, and that really scares you. If you step into your power more and feel more confident in yourself, I think you will be more open and forgiving when things go wrong."

She made the altar, picking images and items that imbued her with a sense of power: Bright yellow candles, amber crystals, and imagery of her favorite saints like Mother Mary and Saint Monica. I suggested using essential oils like ginger, bergamot, ylang-ylang, black pepper, and lavender, which she diluted and used in her bathwater at night. She also burned incense with sandalwood and cedarwood, good for opening the solar plexus.

For movement, I created a solar plexus opening yoga sequence for her, featuring poses like crescent pose, bow pose, boat pose, and plank pose. We wanted her to engage in core-strengthening exercises that would help bring awareness to her seat of power. I also suggested a large foam roller that she lay on once or twice a day. This helped to deeply open her chest and unlock years of pent-up tension in her chest and back.

Something interesting began to happen as we began to release Mercedes's solar plexus. She started to cry—a lot. Almost every day she would find herself sobbing. Of course, she found this very distressing at first. But I assured her this was a very good sign.

"You have a lot to mourn," I told her. "You've never allowed yourself to mourn what you didn't have as a child. You tried to be so strong for so many people, and now it's time to be strong for you . . . and that means feeling all the feelings coming up right now."

She came to agree. Because the more she cried, the less angry she felt. Her chest felt less tight. She wasn't snapping at her family. And miraculously, she found herself reaching out for Frank.

"She just came up and started cuddling the other day," said Frank during a couples' session. "She hasn't hugged me in forever. It was amazing."

Little by little, Mercedes found ways to start owning her personal power, but the first step was realizing that her perception of power had been all wrong. She started to learn the difference between truly being in power versus being in control, which is a mirage in the first place, because no one is truly in control of the universe. But we can be in power with the universe, meaning we can co-create our realities and curate the way we react to things, whether it's a minor traffic delay or a massive trauma.

Frank and Mercedes are still together and still working on healing. They have many years of disconnection to forgive and many layers of love to rebuild, but they're united and willing to do the work. And most importantly, little Mercedes has started to come out again. Despite being fifty-six years old, Mercedes has started letting herself have a second childhood of sorts. She takes vacations to Disneyland every chance she gets, and she has started letting other people take care of her and even baby her when she's having a hard time.

"I was always so scared to need help," she said. "I guess I was scared that the help wouldn't come. That I would be left alone. But that's not what happened. Every time I have let myself be soft and accept help, love just comes pouring in. The other day I had a migraine, and not only did Frank clean the house for me while I napped, but my little brother came over and took my kids to soccer practice. People rally around you if you let them. I never knew that."

Through connection and vulnerability, Mercedes found her strength. And it all started with something as simple as opening her solar plexus chakra!

CHAPTER 4

Erotic Embodiment for Mind-Blowing Sex

> Once you start approaching your body with curiosity rather than with fear, everything shifts . . . Physical self-awareness is the first step in releasing the tyranny of the past.
>
> **—Bessel van der Kolk**

Embodiment can be simply boiled down to one thing: awareness. The present moment is our most powerful tool, and yet we can't wield its power without awareness. Once we bring curiosity to the equation, we feel the world expand. Colors become brighter. Sounds become fuller. We are more in our body and deeply attuned to our feeling senses. Now imagine how that will feel in the bedroom: more awareness plus more sensual feedback equals more pleasure!

UNDERSTANDING EMBODIMENT

When you are embodied, in-your-body, you can feel the full experience of sex, and more fully master the movement of sexual energy within you and between you and a partner. But in addition to this, when you are embodied, your brain and your body are deeply connected and in constant communion. In your daily life, you can connect to the senses, strengthen the bond with your body, and follow your body's wisdom. It is always communicating with you and guiding you, pointing you in the right direction. You just have to listen. When you practice and commit to embodiment, and listen to what your body is telling you, several things happen:

* You become more present in and attuned to the world around you, able to engage all the senses.
* Your ability to experience pleasure and sensuality drastically increases.
* As your body gets the message that you will listen to and follow its guidance, it starts to communicate with you more and more.

RECOGNIZING THE ROLE OF TRAUMA IN EMBODIMENT

In addition to being our guide, and the means to maximum pleasure, our bodies also hold our trauma and losses for us. Our bodies carry our pain even when our minds become distracted or disconnected from our physical selves. We store traumatic experiences in our bodies. In his research on trauma survivors, psychiatrist and post-traumatic stress disorder (PTSD) specialist Bessel van der Kolk found that people with a history of trauma often carry physical side effects from these experiences.

Trauma survivors often cope with their pain by living in a state of disassociation in which they aren't comfortable feeling what is happening inside of their bodies, so they train themselves to essentially become disembodied. In the face of the trauma, many victims learn to shut down the brain areas that accompany and define terror. But by doing so, they also shut themselves off from the entire range of emotions and sensations, which ultimately deadens the capacity to feel fully alive.

You might be thinking, "Well, I never had any real trauma." Let's get a little deeper into the concepts of "Big T, little t" trauma. Trauma can come in many different shapes and forms. "Big T" traumas are the experiences we tend to think about when we think about trauma: war, famine, sexual violence, emotional or physical abuse, and homelessness, for instance.

But "little t" trauma is carried in our bodies in the same way. "Little t" traumas are those experiences that shaped our understanding of the world, our worthiness (or lack thereof), and our expectations of how we would be treated by other people for being our authentic selves.

Some examples of "little t" trauma might be getting bullied in elementary or high school, being criticized or teased about your appearance, growing up in a family with addiction, getting divorced, not being chosen for a sorority, getting cheated on, or getting fired. Painful experiences that scare us, threaten our sense of self, and flood our bodies with cortisol, the stress hormone, can often be "little t" traumas that we continue to carry with us all the time.

The beauty of being with our trauma—by which I mean acknowledging that it exists, holding space for it, allowing it to take whatever form it needs, and attending to it with quiet tenderness and even wonder and gratitude—is that it allows us to honor it and release it. This is even true for the trauma that occurred in our family lineage before we were born.

So many things are passed down in families: heirlooms, physical characteristics, even genetic conditions. But we are now learning that trauma can be inherited as well. This is known as generational trauma (or intergenerational trauma). Scientists have now discovered that trauma affects genetic processes, and can be passed down through epigenetic mechanisms, possibly impacting DNA and gene function.

So not only do we have our "Big T" and "little t" traumas to work through, but we are also carrying with us the trauma of our parents and even past ancestors as well. In addition, generational trauma is passed down when our parents carry their own unresolved trauma and it emerges in their parenting styles. Dysfunctional family dynamics, such as parental emotional immaturity, codependency, unhealthy attachment styles, family stories of traumatic events constantly retold, and regular sharing of memories and photographs of traumatic events are common in these cases.

Regardless of your trauma history, you will always be best supported working with a therapist, coach, or other mental health expert who has experience with trauma healing. This journey is not easy to travel without the help of a trained clinician. Look for someone who is well versed in somatic healing, nervous system retraining, neuro-linguistic reprogramming, sensorimotor psychotherapy, and other forms of integrative psychotherapy.

EXPLORING SOMATIC EXPERIENCING

Somatic Experiencing (SE) has become one of my favorite ways to help myself and the people I counsel to come back to their bodies and move through and heal trauma. It removes the blocks that are holding them back from pleasure. It is a form of therapy that focuses on the body's innate ability to heal from emotional or physical trauma by releasing stored survival energies, such as fight, flight, or freeze responses, that may have become trapped or stuck in the nervous system. By gently guiding individuals to tune into bodily sensations and impulses, SE aims to restore balance and resilience to the nervous system, allowing for a more complete integration of traumatic experiences.

Somatic Experiencing sessions typically involve a combination of somatic awareness exercises, mindfulness techniques, and gentle exploration of traumatic memories and bodily sensations. Through this process, individuals learn to develop greater resilience, self-regulation, and capacity to navigate life's challenges with greater ease and presence.

It's important to note that Somatic Experiencing is often used in conjunction with other therapeutic modalities and should be facilitated by trained and certified practitioners. I often refer people to the website www.traumahealing.org as a resource for finding Somatic Experiencing therapists in their area.

Breathwork and Somatic Experiencing

Breathwork is a form of Somatic Experiencing, based on the understanding that the breath is intimately connected to our physiological and psychological states, and that by altering the way we breathe, we can influence our overall health and consciousness. It encompasses a variety of techniques and practices that focus on conscious manipulation of the breath to promote physical, emotional, and spiritual well-being.

I discovered breathwork when I was working through some of my own trauma, and I was astounded at how profoundly it impacted my ability to feel embodied. I then began teaching my clients about breathwork and including breathwork in the retreats I lead, and I have been so pleased with the results. In addition to feeling more grounded in your body, benefits of breathwork may include stress reduction, improved mental clarity, enhanced emotional resilience, and increased self-awareness.

I find that in addition to its healing effects, breathwork is one of the most effective ways to increase blood flow all over the body (including to your genitals), increase internal sexual and general energy, and activate your nervous system in a calm and empowering way. *Pranayama* is an ancient breathwork technique that aims to regulate the breath for energy cultivation and spiritual development. There are many different pranayama techniques, each with its own benefits and effects. Here's my favorite way to practice pranayama breathwork.

1. Put on some peaceful or inspiring music that takes you inward.
2. Lie down flat on the floor or bed. The key is in keeping your throat area constriction-free. Do not place a pillow under your head.
3. Begin with diaphragmatic breathing, which engages the full capacity of your lungs. Place one hand on your abdomen and the other on your chest. As you inhale deeply through your nose, feel your abdomen expand like a balloon, pushing your hand out. As you exhale, feel your abdomen contract, gently drawing your navel toward your spine. Take five to ten deep breaths to ground yourself.
4. There are many forms of pranayama breath techniques, but for sexual purposes I find the 2-to-1 breath technique most effective. It involves inhaling in two short, powerful sipping breaths through the mouth, almost like you are sucking forcefully through a straw, followed by one longer, forceful exhale through the mouth.

5. If you are new to breathwork, set the timer for ten minutes at first, but ideally work your way up to twenty-five to forty-five minutes. It's important to note that for the first few minutes you will usually meet some internal resistance and want to stop, but keep going. I promise the benefits will be significant. You can even do this alone or with a partner prior to sex to get the blood flowing and your energy centers activated to maximize the sexual experience.

6. After completing your breathwork practice, take a few moments to observe any changes in your body, mind, and breath. Notice how you feel physically, mentally, and emotionally.

Note that you may experience tingling in your body or extremities, increased heart rate, cramping, lightheadedness (which is why it's extra helpful to be lying down), or an emotional release. Just let it all flow as it needs to. If you get cramping in your hands or feet, it's usually a sign of blocked energy wanting to move. It helps to imagine that the soles of your feet or palms of your hands have energetic portals in them. As you breathe out, imagine the energy moving through them.

KEEPING AN EMBODIMENT JOURNAL

One of my favorite ways to help my clients become more consciously embodied and notice where they may be unconsciously leaving or disassociating from their bodies is by keeping a record of their daily experience of their body and their senses. Most of us run through our days on autopilot, barely attuning to our bodies unless we are hungry, in pain, or experiencing some other physical need. Numerous studies have suggested that regularly keeping a gratitude journal can increase overall feelings of gratitude and general well-being. This is in large part because when you keep a gratitude journal, the lens through which you are experiencing your life changes because you are looking for—and therefore noticing—things for which you feel grateful.

The embodiment journal works the same way. As you set the intention to notice when you are in your body and feel the sensations there, you begin to spend more and more time in your body. It doesn't have to be complicated. You can even keep a list on your smartphone. Just keep a record when you notice a sensation that triggers your senses, like a beautiful smell or the feeling of the breeze on your skin. Set the intention to make five entries a day, even if it's at the end of the day going back over the sensory experiences you've had.

WORKING TOWARD EROTIC EMBODIMENT

Erotic embodiment involves the grounding of the erotic expression of the soul and the sensations of erotic arousal within the body in a way that you can feel.

To achieve erotic embodiment, we must become embodied, or in the body. Most of us aren't fully in our bodies during the day and we aren't even in our bodies during sex. In fact, sex might be the most difficult place for you to become embodied.

While erotic embodiment might sound like a beautiful, healing process, it is also important to note that you might find it a little triggering or overwhelming. That's because your body is very wise and compassionate. It is looking out for you, all the time, even when you don't realize it. Somewhere along the line, being *in* your body felt really scary or distressing or even traumatic. So you disengaged from it. Your senses dulled. You pulled inward, almost as if you were watching yourself in third person instead of actually being in your own person.

It is difficult to become fully embodied in the bedroom until you are able to begin to work through what sent you under the bed in the first place—and what is still keeping you there.

You don't have to do it all at once. And if you have significant trauma, I wouldn't advise that you try to do this without the help of a therapist. But trust the process. Think of it like doing a deep-clean of your house: At first, things look worse as you start pulling things out of drawers and lifting up the couch cushions. But over time, each mess gets tackled and organized. You begin to feel lighter. More in control. More capable of confronting the next mess.

Please begin this process with your safety and well-being in mind. Don't push yourself to a breaking point. Listen to your body and notice when things become overwhelming. I want these exercises to trigger growth, not trauma.

Exercises to Access Embodiment

Let's start with a few exercises geared at figuring out how you became erotically disembodied. Find a spot that offers quiet and privacy, whether it is your bedroom or your favorite spot at a local park.

Look back at the first physical sensations you can recall as a child. I know, this is going to be strange at first. But I don't want you to think only of your first memories. I want you to think of how you physically felt in your body during those memories. Here are some examples from my clients over the years:

* I remember playing on the beach with my older sister. The sun was so hot, and the sand almost burned our feet. The waves were cold, and we screamed as we ran in and out of the tides. My sides hurt from laughing so much.

SEX MAGIC

* I remember being whipped with a belt. I can feel the leather on my skin and my mother's fingers roughly holding me around the arm like a vise. I want to throw up. I can't breathe. My fear is making me shake uncontrollably.

* I remember rolling out challah dough with my grandmother. Her kitchen was so warm from her old stove. The room smelled yeasty and slightly sweet, like her perfume was lingering in the air. I remember feeling the dough, soft and pliant between my fingers, and feeling Nana's warm, dry hands over mine as she taught me how to braid it.

* I remember watching my parents argue in the living room. I am hiding behind the recliner. I can feel the corduroy fabric against my cheek. I am trying to be so small. My hands are covering my ears. I can smell the oil on my father's coveralls. My chest feels tight. The air conditioner vent is blowing cool air on my bare legs. Outside I can hear the neighbor kids playing in the front yard. I hope they can't hear my parents.

Now, I need to offer a caveat: Whenever I first ask my clients to start recalling their first memories with these intimate physical details, they don't come to them easily. Instead, they would recall memories like "I remember getting beat with a belt," or "I remember my parents yelling and how scary and embarrassing it was." Or "I remember baking with my granny," or "I remember being on the beach with my sister."

But as part of becoming embodied in these memories, we work on not just recalling the facts as we remember them, but also the way those experiences *felt*. It will take a few moments to shift into that past version of yourself, but once you do, you might be surprised at how quickly you can not only recall those old physical sensations but at how much you can start to feel them in the present.

This can be really unpleasant if you're recalling a traumatic memory. That is why I advise you first start by trying to source the physical sensations of happy memories. It will help create that feel-good serotonin boost and make you more excited to try this exercise again, rather than turning it into something you might fear.

The body remembers and keeps the score of our "Big T" and "little t" trauma, but it also keeps the score of our most precious experiences as well. Think of your most sacred memories, the memories etched in your heart for all time. Perhaps you're thinking of when you held your baby for the first time. Your child might be an adult by now, but I bet that memory feels like a physical spark inside your chest. You might feel your heart physically clench or your arms tighten as you remember the soft, warm weight of the baby's body. That memory is living in you, both emotionally and physically.

Maybe you're thinking of your first crush at junior prom. You can probably still feel the butterflies and the thrill of excitement in your body. Or maybe you're thinking of sitting in your grandma's kitchen, having tea and helping her make cookies. Even if it's been years since you entered that space, years since your grandmother was alive, you can physically feel yourself in that kitchen, can't you? You can feel the heat of the stove, the heft of the teacup in your small hands, her love buoying you up like a fantastic tidal wave.

Every stride you take toward embodiment is going to be felt and appreciated by your body. The body keeps score but the body also forgives. The universe is arced toward healing. It is not rigged against you. It is working with you. And the secret lies in embodiment, because once we master that, we can then master learning to move with the universe's harmonic waves.

WORKING THROUGH THE ENERGETIC HANGOVER OF SEX

Just like when you wake up with a hangover after a rough night out, you can wake up with a hangover when you're having sex that is not in line with your heart and mind. You might think casual sex is no big deal, but you're taking on more than just physical risks, like STIs and unwanted pregnancy.

Every time you have sex, you are opening your body up to receive the energy of the person you are with. This is especially true if you are an empath and even more so if you are a woman. Yes, female empaths, this is a double whammy for you! You are a powerful vessel for receiving energy, and yet you must be thoughtful about what energy you are allowing into your body, because this energy will not necessarily leave just because your hookup walks out the door.

When you are in an embodied state, you will be fully in your power when you decide who to share your body with, and you will be much less likely to wake up with a nasty energetic sex hangover.

Use Your Heart Chakra to Protect Your Energetic Body

You learned about the heart chakra and the green, beautiful, eternal flame in the center in chapter 3. There is a next level to which you can take the eternal flame of your heart that serves to keep you protected from negative energies around you. And it can keep you from being affected by other people's energy.

Our energetic states are contagious. And the more *in* our bodies we are, the more we can feel it when we are holding energy states that are out of alignment. This is part of why it's hard for you when your partner comes home in a bad mood, even if they act perfectly kind to you.

EROTIC EMBODIMENT FOR MIND-BLOWING SEX

It's also why you may find yourself feeling out of sorts after spending time with someone or have a "bad feeling" for no apparent reason about someone you just met. These aren't just gut feelings; they are often your body reading the energy around you. And very often we get jangly and agitated inside our bodies when exposed to the energy of others, especially those in low-frequency states.

Here's a simple and fast way to create an energetic field of protection around you. It's wonderful to do this in the morning at the start of the day, when you are about to walk into a situation with a lot of other people, or when you are going to be spending time with someone you know tends to be manipulative or negative.

1. Follow steps 1–5 from the heart chakra's eternal flame exercise you learned in chapter 3 (sit or lie quietly, do a body scan, focus on building the small powerful flame in the center of your heart chakra, and let it get brighter and brighter). But this time, instead of radiating the energy out into the world, ask the energy you've been building inside you to expand out of your body to create a bubble surrounding you. With each breath, envision it spreading out a little further, until you have created a bubble of light around you that surrounds your entire being, four feet in every direction.

2. You can say out loud or to yourself, "This bubble is a filter. Only that energy which is aligned with the highest frequency of love is allowed in, and only that which I choose to release is allowed out. And so it is."

3. I also like to infuse my bubble with light from the violet flame. This is the light of the Holy Spirit, pure and protective. It burns away all that doesn't serve and protect you. As you sit in the energy of your bubble, envision violet light showering

down over your bubble and, with your permission, permeating the filter. Let the beautiful, sparkling violet light fill the bubble and surround you in the violet flame. Ask it to burn away anything that doesn't serve and transmute it to love.

To intentionally clear anyone's (or anything's) energy from my field, I love to use this exercise:

1. After grounding, with your eyes still closed, envision a beautiful rose a couple of feet in front of you.
2. The rose is the most purifying vacuum you can imagine. Envision the rose sucking all the energy that isn't yours off your field. It might help to see the stuff coming off you as a color or texture (green and gooey or brown and slick, for instance).
3. You can imagine the rose traveling slowly over the front and back of your body, even over your head and under your feet.
4. When you feel satisfied that all that is currently "on you" is off, you can blow up the rose. Envision it exploding into a million bits and pieces, each of them being pulled up into the sky, transforming into pure light.
5. You can say (out loud or silently): "All that has been removed isn't mine; it doesn't serve me or anyone else to carry it. I am releasing all that the rose has absorbed back to Oneness (Spirit, God, Universe, whatever you wish to say), to be transmuted to love."

Sexual Healing Meditation

So what do you do with that energetic hangover from past sexual partners, especially those who hurt you? Sexual healing is ultimately

EROTIC EMBODIMENT FOR MIND-BLOWING SEX

about releasing the energetic remains of past hurts or traumas related to your body or your sexuality. This could have been times when you were mistreated or hurt during or after a sexual encounter. It could be the need to release a past relationship that was toxic or abusive.

Despite the traumas you may have suffered—and whether or not the people who harmed you were ever held accountable—you can rest confidently in the knowledge that sexual healing is yours to claim.

I have worked with so many people whose sexual power and pleasure are limited due to past hurts, humiliations, rejections, or traumas. I created a sexual healing kit and meditation to help release the negative energy of the past. You can listen to a guided version of this meditation at drlauraberman.com/sexmagic.

To experience the meditation, you will need:

* A candle (pillar or jar)
* Palo santo or sage: These powerful herbs are known for their clarifying and cleansing properties. Find them at your natural foods store or online.
* Rose quartz wand: Rose quartz is believed to carry the vibration of love and help absorbs negative energy. You can find these online. Make sure to energetically clean it before use by bathing it in Himalayan pink salt and water overnight, or you can put it outside under a full moon overnight as well.
* Bath salts: Choose a kind that is natural and chemical-free.

This is a process of energetic release and sexual healing. The goal is to relax into it and let go in a healing and safe way. The exercise is ideally done in the bathtub, but if you don't have access to a bath, you can do this meditation without the bath salts and the bath. Here are the steps:

SEX MAGIC

1. Set aside twenty to thirty minutes alone where you will have privacy and a safe space. While not mandatory, it will be very helpful to have at least another thirty minutes afterward to integrate the healing and come back into reality.

2. Run the bath with very warm to hot water and pour in your sexual healing bath salts. Smell the fragrance. Activate your senses.

3. Light a candle and set this sacred intention: "I'm lighting this candle to manifest healing, open hardheartedness, space for healing, letting go of the old and that which no longer serves me, and letting in the new."

4. Light some palo santo or sage, gently blowing out the flame so the tip is smoking. Go around the bathroom gently waving the stick so the smoke drifts up into all corners of the room. Say out loud, "I'm creating a safe container of healing. The only energy that comes into the room will be the energy aligned with love, acceptance, and healing."

5. Stand in the bathroom and ground yourself. Imagine a beautiful light, any color you want, coming in through the top of your head and moving down through your tailbone and deep into the Earth. Do that at least three times while taking deep breaths. Your rose quartz healing wand has already been cleared of all other energies and it's safe to use.

6. Enter the bath with the rose quartz wand. Rest. Enjoy the scent of the water. Notice how it feels on your skin. Remember to attune to your senses. Allow that sensual awareness to build, being in your body.

7. When you are ready, place the rose quartz wand on your heart, on your belly, or if you feel ready, you can insert it into your vagina or anus, depending on where you want to focus

the healing. You can hold it there or release the hold and let it rest inside. As you do so, allow your body to relax. Notice the sensations that you may or may not feel. Invite the wand to absorb all that you want to let go of, all the negative energy of the past—all the times your boundaries were not respected, all the energy that you no longer want to hold and is blocking your divine feminine. Allow the rose quartz to transmute it all to love.

8. Whenever you are ready and as often as you wish, remove the healing wand. There is no right or wrong way of doing this, just follow your heart and your instincts.

9. When finished with the meditation, allow yourself some time to decompress. Make sure you clear your wand after each use by soaking it overnight, preferably under the Moon, in sea salt mixed with warm water.

Sexual Healing through Conscious Penile Penetration

If you are in a safe, loving relationship with a partner who has a penis, you can use penetration, not only to create more intensity and pleasure between you, but to create healing. Thanks to somatic therapies, it is now in our Western understanding that the body stores painful memories and emotions, including in the vagina and entire pelvic region.

In the Tantric tradition, the head of the penis is considered a powerful healing force that can act as a magnet with the power to remove or transmute old memories or pain that is energetically stored inside the partner. At the same time, the feminine is considered most receptive to energetic healing and release in the deepest parts of her vagina, the cervix and the base of the uterus. Healing through penetration requires trust.

Here's how it works.

1. Make a plan with your partner around your intention for healing through penetration. You don't even have to know exactly what you want to heal; just setting that intention is enough.
2. Create a soft and safe nest for your healing penetration: soft music, comfy blankets, and perhaps some candles.
3. Ground yourself and get present in your body.
4. Because this is an exercise in building healing energy between you, it is not necessary to engage in a lot of foreplay or treat this as a typical sexual encounter. An erection is not necessary, but is fine if it happens.
5. After lubricating the penis and the vaginal entrance, gently spread the labia apart as the head of the penis is gently placed right at the entrance.
6. Wait a few moments and then enter slowly, stopping every half inch or so, taking some deep slow breaths, then entering in another half inch.
7. There is no thrusting, just gentle incremental insertion of the penis into the vagina. It is important not to use lots of pressure against the walls of the vagina, as this might cause the vaginal muscles to tighten and resist.
8. Continue penetration slowly, inch by inch, taking several deep breaths in between, until the penis feels some resistance against the head. This is when the penis is usually touching the cervix or the top end of the vagina. Pull back just a fraction to create more space for the magnetic penis head to create a field of energetic polarity with the cervix.

9. It is important that if any pain is experienced this is immediately communicated and the penis should pull back. Pain often is a sign of old memories or trauma held in the tissue. Or there may be pain in the penis, testicles, or groin. Just hold the penis in that area for several moments to see what occurs; there may be sensations of throbbing, pulsing, or even stinging. Sometimes sadness or fear may rise to the surface. There is no need to interpret or analyze what is coming up at this point. The idea is to hold all the emotions that emerge with reverence and honor them as part of the purification and healing process. Just allow the feelings to pass through while you hold each other gently and keep breathing.

10. Over time the goal is for the penis to explore and touch all angles and spaces in the vagina, which will soften and yield as healing and a sense of safety increases.

BECOMING FULLY EMBODIED TO ENHANCE SEX

Can you think of a time when you felt fully embodied during sex? Or maybe just during a sensual act or self-stimulating? By "fully embodied," I mean fully in your body, attuned to your senses and not losing time or focus. Some people might not be able to recall feeling embodied during sex, but they might vividly remember how physically in tune they felt when they were making out with their high school crush. Can you recall a time like that? A time when you felt like you were in the flow and your body and your spirit were in harmony and fully present?

Maybe that's only ever happened to you in the yoga studio or while you're on a long run or a bike ride. Maybe you felt it on the field when you were on the college baseball team, or perhaps when you were creating in the art studio.

It's almost hard to describe how it feels to be embodied, but you can easily describe it when you aren't, can't you? You know when you feel a million miles away from yourself. Maybe you're an introvert who gets so dysregulated by big social events that it takes you days to return to yourself after the holidays. Maybe you go into survival mode when you're around a certain family member and you can literally feel yourself disappear when that triggering person is around.

What does it feel like to be embodied? Think of a few words or phrases that you can use to describe that feeling of being home in your body. Maybe even write them down.

Here's how my clients describe their experiences with embodiment:

* Perfect rhythm
* Supercharged
* Like I'm surfing and the wave never breaks
* Blissed out
* Powerful and competent
* Purring like a cat
* Lit up from the inside out, glowing all over

This is how my clients describe *dis*embodiment:

* Fuzzy, like an old TV on a dead channel
* Can't hear myself think
* Remote. Lonely.
* Numb, like the world is going on around me, but through a glass wall
* Constipated. Stuck. Powerless.

EROTIC EMBODIMENT FOR MIND-BLOWING SEX

* Like my cheeks hurt from fake smiling
* Distracted, forgetful, everything is moving too fast

Did those examples help you to get into the zone? Remember, there are no right or wrong answers. Literally anything you think is the right answer. Learning to trust yourself to think is actually a really key part of becoming embodied, because if you don't trust yourself and you're always second-guessing yourself, you get caught up in a rumination cycle. And it's downright impossible to ruminate and catastrophize and be embodied all the same time.

So let trusting your answers be part of this exercise. No one else can answer this but you, and no one else is more expert than you in this field. This is your domain. Own it!

Once you have made your lists, read them both over. You likely didn't feel embodied because you are a size zero or because your penis is huge. You didn't feel embodied because you were wearing expensive lingerie or because your house was immaculate and everything on your to-do list was marked off.

Here are some of the most effective ways I find I am able to help people to come back to their bodies when they have a trauma history or a history of disassociating from their bodies.

Enhance the Senses to Build Erotic Embodiment

You can't engage in sex magic if you don't take your body seriously. If you don't treat your body with dignity, curiosity, and reverence, your sex life is going to suffer. Part of becoming erotically embodied is realizing that your body isn't some strange vessel that is not associated with your soul or your mind.

Humans tend to suffer from the belief that the physical isn't as important as the emotional. Because we can think and ponder and make amazing inventions, we think that the brain is superior to the body. In fact, we say this all the time: It's what's on the inside that matters. Or beauty is only skin-deep. Or it's the soul that counts.

But something really amazing happens when we stop viewing our body as a separate entity and start living like our bodies matter. And I don't mean the way your body *looks* because that has nothing to do with your body. Those are other people's expectations and our culture's ideals.

I mean living like your body's experience matters. Like your body has wisdom for you and mysteries for you to unfold. Like your senses aren't just how you navigate the external world, but part of how you navigate your inner world as well. Think of a cat's whiskers or a dog's nose: Animals live and die by the information they get from their senses. All wild things do. And, at our core, that is all that we are. Our bodies evolved to give us the best chance at survival in this world and required more than just cognition. It required us to become uniquely tactile creatures who could use our senses to run from danger, to find family, and to build community.

Honoring your body's messages and reuniting with your body as a *sacred* part of you means more than just ceasing negative self-talk or harmful activities like smoking. It means relearning how to live *in* your body instead of just with it.

You can try to experiment with this by turning off all the lights in your home at night .Just make sure you don't have any trip hazards so that you don't get hurt. As the darkness floods your senses, notice what happens inside of you. Suddenly you start to feel very inside of your body. You can literally hear your heartbeat in your ears. You can feel your fingers moving through the air and the planks of the floor beneath your feet. Isn't it funny how instantly we can become in our bodies when we just take away the light for a moment?

If you feel safe and you don't have any mobility issues, you can try walking around a little bit. Use the walls as your guide as you move around. Notice how different your house sounds or even smells in the dark. Can you imagine being in a cave millions of years ago with your ancestors? How did they have to use their bodies to survive? How did they learn to rely on their bodies' messages when they didn't have a fire, much less a flashlight or light switches to show their path?

If you don't feel comfortable doing this exercise while walking around, you can also do it while sitting in the bathtub. Run a warm bubble bath and turn off the lights. Sink into the water slowly and notice how differently you experience even the most ordinary thing like a bar of soap. The world becomes louder and quieter all at once. You hear everything and you feel everything and yet you let go of things more readily. You're seeking for what matters, what physical messages are important for your safety and well-being. There are no thoughts of your cellulite or the soap scum you missed when you cleaned earlier.

If you have a partner, you can start playing with the senses together. Try having sex with a blindfold on, or without making any sounds. I know this sounds like the opposite of sexy. After all, having sex with the lights on and communicating during sex are things I often recommend!

But if you're struggling with being disembodied, sex in pitch darkness can be so helpful, especially if you're neurodivergent. It can remove all those distractions and keep you hyper-focused on what is happening in the moment.

The same is true for having a silent session. How can you communicate with each other if you can't use words? How can you pleasure each other if you must "listen" to each other's bodies instead of your words? You can even role-play that you don't want someone to hear you or that you must be super-quiet because you're in public. However you decide to do it, just remember that I am asking you to be quiet and in the dark not because I want you to turn off your senses, but because you are learning to turn them back *on*.

Notice how much more closely you have to pay attention to your partner's little clues, such as their breathing or their heartbeat. Are you more able to notice your own arousal as well? Do you feel more in your body? What feelings do you notice physically?

As you can see, creating sex magic is about more than just the spiritual realm. Having sacred, meaningful sex doesn't mean that we don't include our material selves—just the opposite. Every part of you belongs. Every part of you can be seen and honored in the bedroom.

Medibate to Open the Energy Channels for Amazing Sex

How about creating meaningful sex with yourself? Medibation involves masturbation (alone or with a partner) that is done as a conscious meditation. It is not about arousal or orgasm, although that can often happen.

Medibation is intended to be an intimate practice that enhances sensuality and intimacy, helping you create a bridge between sex and the quantum field, and leading to heightened sensations and stronger energetic awareness. It's a beautiful meditation that feels really wonderful. The key is in the restraint, not falling into usual masturbation patterns, but following the directions. I would suggest doing medibation alone first.

Once you have the hang of it, you can practice with and even teach a partner. You will need privacy, quiet, some candles and soft music, cozy pillows and blankets should you wish, a timer, and a good lubricant.

As far as lubricants go, I am a fan of organic coconut oil (the kind you would cook with), assuming you aren't allergic to coconuts! Otherwise, any organic lubricant will do.

1. Create a medibation nest and gather all the necessary supplies: cozy blankets, pillows, and lubrication. Maybe you want to light some candles or put on some peaceful, meditative music.

2. Get completely undressed and, once comfortable, ground yourself and open your heart. Begin by breathing in for the count of four and breathe out for the count of six for three minutes. Do this while thinking of something or someone for whom you feel uncomplicated love and appreciation. The image you choose need not have anything to do with sex or even a partner. This combination of breath and visualization puts your body into a gentle state of coherence and relaxation.

3. Now set a timer for ten to fifteen minutes. From this coherent and grounded place, apply your lubrication to the genitals and begin gently stroking the clitoris and labia or penis. Use just one or two fingers. Start with a downward stroke in gentle repetitive motions. Remember, this isn't about going to your usual masturbation technique, nor is the goal arousal or orgasm. No internal stimulation. It is all external stroking. Start on one side and then the other.

4. As you stroke yourself gently, begin taking conscious, slow breaths, in through the nose and out through the mouth, timing the in-breaths and out-breaths to your stroking (either one long breath or a couple of shorter deep breaths). A comfortable pace for most is breathing in for one to two slow strokes

and breathing out for one to two slow strokes. You can pause your breath for a stroke in between in-breaths and out-breaths if you wish.

5. Once you get into a rhythm you can begin to change directions with an upward stroke, but continue gentle stroking up and/or down. This is not a time to start circling or putting too much pressure on your stroking.

6. Now that you are in a rhythm of synchronized breathing and stroking, imagine beautiful red, sparkling light coming in from deep in the Earth through the vaginal opening, anus, or the perineum as you breathe in. As you breathe out, let the light circle around your pelvis and become even brighter and deeper in color. Keep repeating; on the in-breath the beautiful red light flows up and in from the center of the Earth as you keep slowly stroking, and on the out breath it circles and intensifies.

7. Continue this stroking, breathing in the light until the timer alerts you to stop. While doing so, stay in touch with your body. What are you noticing? Is there sensation? Arousal? Is it building or staying the same? Is it spreading or changing with the out-breath or in-breath? This is where you can start attuning to the subtle movement of sexual energy in your body, something we will be building on in the exercises later on.

Soft, Slow Sex for Embodiment and Pleasure

With slow sex, instead of focusing on climax or intense passion, you engage in the sexual experience by stepping back, coming fully into your body, and witnessing yourself. In fact, sexual arousal or even foreplay is not necessary in slow sex. So instead of "heating things up" with excitement, you are falling back fully into your body (and your

EROTIC EMBODIMENT FOR MIND-BLOWING SEX

partner into theirs), with no goal, no place to be but together. Slow sex is a practice that can deepen your connection, generating love and harmony between you. Neither arousal nor erection are necessary for slow sex; that's part of the reason it's also considered "soft." Slow sex begins before or without an erection. Consciousness and vitality are the keys, as opposed to excitement and arousal. I find that couples who practice slow sex regularly have a deeper bond, trust, and love and playfulness between them.

1. Give yourselves at least an hour. Remember this is slow sex, not something you are going to fit into a busy schedule. Everything is approached with ease and relaxation.

2. You are together, but also each inwardly focused on your own experience, and not caught up in making sex into a hot, steamy, exciting endeavor. Root yourself in your own body. Picture your spine as a sexual rod or midline running through your system and carrying energy.

3. The easiest position for slow sex is the larger (or masculine) partner lying on their side facing their partner, while the smaller (or feminine) partner lies on their back, their legs intertwined like scissors. If practicing with a male or person with a penis, the penis can be soft during slow sex.

4. Lubricate the genitals with organic lubrication and move your genitals close together. From here, the feminine can take the penis in her two hands and pull down the shaft toward the root of the penis, pulling back any foreskin. Then make a peace sign with both hands. With one hand (typically the left), place the base of the penis between the forefinger and middle finger and gently squeeze so you have a firm grip and pull the penis. Place the peace fingers of the other hand right

below the head of the penis and begin gently pulling the penis (with both hands) toward the vaginal or anal opening.

5. When the head of the penis is close to the vaginal opening, begin gently pushing the penis a little way into the vagina or anus. Pull the fingers back a little and feed the penis farther and farther into the vaginal opening, until you have pushed the entire length of the penis into the vagina. Don't worry if it's awkward at first or you can get only a little bit of the penis inside. It gets much easier with practice.

6. When insertion is complete, wrap your legs around one another. Relax all your muscles, especially the anus and buttocks, and tune into your bodies.

7. There is no need to move or thrust. Eyes are open and receptive. Smile at each other. Talk to one another with love. Notice what happens. A spontaneous erection or arousal may occur and that's fine; just embrace the slowness. Detach from the orgasmic goal. This is about intimacy and connection, and each of you deeply, internally experiencing the energy of your slow sexual penetration.

Tune into the Kegels and Pelvic Floor to Maximize Pleasure

You experimented with your Kegels already in chapter 3 with the Chakra Elevator exercise. Let's take a deeper dive into these important muscles. Your Kegels are the muscles that surround the anus and vagina or scrotum in a figure-eight pattern. The male pelvic floor supports the bladder and the bowels, and it also plays a key role in their sexual function. The female pelvic floor supports the bladder and bowels, but it has the additional role of supporting the uterus.

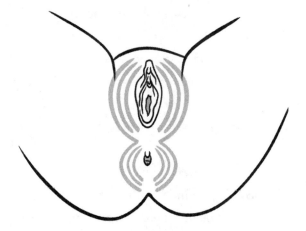

Kegel muscles in the female

As its name suggests, the pelvic floor is a floor, or hammock of muscles, at the base of our pelvis. You might have also heard it called "the floor of the core," which is a helpful way to visualize it. The pelvic floor is composed of muscles, ligaments, nerves, and fascia. Our pelvic floor works in tandem with the deepest layer of our abdominal muscles. Our transversus abdominus contracts alongside our pelvic floor. That is why if you have a weak core, you might experience symptoms related to your bowel or bladder, because these muscles work in tandem. A strong pelvic floor and a strong core go hand in hand.

You can identify and isolate your Kegels by squeezing and releasing the muscles you use to stop and start urine flow. Don't exercise them while urinating because that can lead to a urinary tract infection. You can identify and strengthen your pelvic floor by doing any kind of "core" exercise.

Remember, while Kegels can help tighten and strengthen your muscles to improve both vaginal tone and sexual performance, the true benefit is that you are consciously sending breath and awareness to this area, bringing awareness and embodiment to your genitals. Most of all, use of the Kegels and the pelvis are central to moving sexual energy. The stronger and more flexible those muscles are, the more easily you can propel genital sensation up and around your body, and between you and your partner.

Here are my top tips for effective Kegel exercises:

* Slow and steady always wins the race—no, scratch that, there is no race! Don't aim to do twenty or thirty reps as fast as you can. Be thoughtful and intentional. Go slowly. Breathe. Squeeze. Hold. Breathe. Release. Repeat. And repeat. If you want to use Kegel weights or pelvic floor exercisers, apply the same logic. You shouldn't try to get the heaviest weight or the most intense exerciser. Slow and low is the tempo. That is going to get into those slow-twitch muscle fibers that are the powerhouses of the core.

* Try diaphragmatic breathing (also explained in chapter 4). Place one hand on your abdomen and the other on your chest, inhaling deeply through your nose, feel your abdomen expand like a balloon pushing your hand out. As you exhale, feel your abdomen contract, gently drawing your navel toward your spine. You can strengthen your core and your pelvic floor with these deep belly breaths. You want to engage your deepest core muscles to create this breath. Lie flat on the ground with your knees bent. Make sure your back is well supported on the floor without an arch. Your lower back should be flush with the floor. Now, place one hand on your chest and one hand on your lower belly. Breathe in through your nose and feel the air extending down to the basement of your core. The

EROTIC EMBODIMENT FOR MIND-BLOWING SEX

hand on your belly should rise from this inhale, but not the hand on your chest. Now, slowly but forcefully release that breath. Again, your chest should not be moving. This is deep belly breathing. It may be very difficult to do at first. Most of us take quite shallow breaths out of habit, and we don't know how to get breath deep out of our belly or put breath back into our belly. But it can be incredibly powerful for your core, as well as very relaxing and restorative.

* Don't forget anal Kegels. Like I said, your pelvic floor also supports your bowels. Use the muscles that you would use to stop and start a bowel movement or gas. Squeeze and release these muscles just as you would for regular Kegel exercises, where you imagine stopping the flow of urine.

* Try simple yoga positions to engage and strengthen the pelvic floor. Here are some of my favorite yoga positions for pelvic floor engagement:

    * Boat pose: Arrange yourself on your sit bones on a comfortable floor or yoga mat with your legs stretched out in front of you. Use your core muscles to lift your legs in front of you, a few inches off the floor. Extend your arms in front of you at the same time. Use your core muscles to hold yourself in this pose, using your deepest ab muscles to support your body in the air.

    * Cat-cow: Get on all fours. Engage the ab muscles to gently lift your lower abs up to the sky. (Picture the silhouette of a Halloween cat.) Your back should gently rise in such a manner. But it is not the back that is doing the lifting; you are using your ab muscles to lift your belly upward. Then release, allowing the belly to gently sag

into cow pose. Do a few reps between cat-cow, breathing deeply and moving thoughtfully as you isolate these deep ab muscles.

* Reclined pelvic twist: This is great if your pelvic floor is tight or restricted. It can help to break up some of that fascia in your pelvis and keeps things open and flexible. Like any muscle, the vagina needs to be flexible, pliable, and active. It needs to be able to contract and *relax*. A reclining pelvic floor twist is a great pose to help us get deep in the core and get out some tension in our pelvic floor. Lie flat on your back with your arms extended out in a T shape. Then gently lift and twist your hips over to the right side so that you are bent at the knees but still firm and flat on the ground. You will feel a beautiful, deep stretch in your lower back, but it is also breaking up that pelvic floor fascia and getting blood moving down there.

CONNECTING WITH YOUR BODY THROUGH ECSTATIC DANCE

Ecstatic dancing is a unique form of dance that is free-form and spontaneous, prioritizing self-expression and self-discovery. It is ancient, with roots in various spiritual and cultural traditions around the world, such as tribal dancing, shamanic rituals, and Sufi whirling. Many who practice ecstatic dance experience it as transformative.

If you want to connect more to your body and feel the energies running through it, I highly recommend playing with ecstatic dance. I can tell you the first time I tried it I didn't know what to expect, but after one session I was hooked. I loved the rush of feel-good chemicals ecstatic dancing created in my body and I experienced it as bringing me back into my body better than almost anything else I tried. I also loved the way the dancing moved-pent up energy out of my body, especially any anger or grief I was unintentionally holding in.

You don't have to be coordinated or even a decent dancer. You just must be willing to suspend thinking as much as you can, and let your body take the lead, moving the way it wants. Ecstatic dancing is typically done in a group setting, but even in groups most people are in their own worlds dancing on their own.

How to Practice Ecstatic Dance

Are you are ready to try ecstatic dancing? There are three ways to explore it.

Try dancing in an organized group setting. You can find announcements for organizations doing ecstatic dance experiences on local community bulletin boards in places like yoga studios or community centers.

You can also create your own ecstatic dance event with friends or family. All you need is some great dance music and some space in which to move freely. You can blast the music on a speaker or let everyone tap into your playlist with their own headphones.

One of the most common ways to experience ecstatic dancing is to have your own private dance party. I highly recommend this regardless of what organized ecstatic dancing you do. All you have to do is put on music and dance like no one is watching!

Here are the steps:

1. Set aside a decent amount of time. Ecstatic dance sessions can be ten minutes to three hours! If you're by yourself, you can try dancing for just a few songs at first. However, the idea is to

give yourself enough time to really get into it and let yourself go, so the longer the better.

2. If you are dancing alone (or leading an ecstatic dance session), make sure you have a playlist set up, ideally with numerous songs of different speeds you love. You want to start off slowly and make sure to warm up and loosen up, then the music should get faster and more intense, finally slowing down again toward the end of your session.

3. Create your own playlist of music that inspires you or sets you free. Include slow songs to start, then slowly increase the pace, followed by something even quicker. If you'd like, you can try one of the ecstatic dance mixes I've created myself at drlauraberman.com/sexmagic.

4. Dress comfortably. Wear loose, comfortable clothing that allows for unrestricted movement. Barefoot dancing is usually encouraged, especially if dancing outside, but some people prefer soft dance shoes or socks.

5. Prepare mentally. Before starting, take a few moments to center yourself. Set an intention for your dance session, whether it's to let go of stress, express emotions, or simply have fun.

6. Let yourself go and dance freely. Focus on the music and see if you can suspend any self-consciousness and move however you feel compelled to move. It's normal to be a little self-conscious at first. But what you will discover, even dancing in a group, is that everyone is in their own world, and no one is looking at you! There are no right or wrong moves in ecstatic dancing, so the idea is to trust your instincts and express yourself without judgment.

7. Pay attention to the music's rhythm and flow. Ecstatic dance sessions often include a wide range of genres, from world

music and electronic beats to ambient sounds. Let the music guide your movements.

8. Be mindful of your body. Stay in tune with your body's signals. Take breaks when needed, hydrate, and don't push yourself too hard. The goal is to enjoy the experience without strain.

9. Cool down. As the session comes to an end, gradually slow your movements, and return to a state of stillness. Take a moment to reflect on your experience and how you feel.

10. Share and connect. Some ecstatic dance sessions may end with a circle where participants share their experiences or engage in group activities like hugging or deep breathing.

SEX MAGIC CASE FILE

Zuby is a forty-five-year-old radiologist and mother of three. She was used to always having the answers or being able to find them, even if it took weeks of research. So when I asked her to describe to me a time that she felt embodied and she couldn't, I could tell she felt very frustrated. She wanted to have the "right" answer and complete the assignment.

Zuby grew up in a very traditional, religious household in which her father ruled with an iron fist. Due to her religion, she had to dress very conservatively. She also had to follow very conservative and rigid social customs. She was only very rarely allowed to be a child and play, especially in public, where she was taught not to draw attention to herself. So, in helping her source a time that she felt embodied, we had her look back to her childhood to find those rare moments where she felt free, safe, and away from restrictions.

She came to me with a sudden answer: tennis.

The one place she could be free was at her weekly tennis lessons at her all-girls elementary school. During those lessons, she got to be silly and hang out with her girlfriends, playing in the sun and goofing off. The only problem was that she wasn't very good at tennis. She tried, but it was like she just couldn't do what the other girls did. She mimicked their physical actions. She lobbed the ball across the net. She ran up and down the court sweating under her headwrap. She whacked her racket at any ball that came near her.

Zuby seemed like she was getting worse, not better, as the lessons wore on. She could feel her teacher's frustration with her.

"He thought I was deliberately not trying," she told me. "But what's funny is I was trying so hard it made my brain hurt!"

She hated feeling like her teacher didn't like her. Finally, though, she gave up trying to please him.

"I was always the best student in my grade, the most obedient kid," she said. "So it really drove me nuts that he didn't think I was good. Because it felt just like that: like I wasn't good. Not just at tennis. But all of me."

Then something interesting happened. She got so angry with herself that she just quit. Not the team, because she loved being with her friends. But she decided to quit trying. She wasn't going to whack at every ball. She wasn't going to race like a fool all over the court. She wasn't going to mimic the other girls who were naturals.

She shut everything out but what her coach was saying in the moment. She could feel her attention narrowing and her senses heightening. Suddenly her body wasn't lobbing and racing and whacking. She was flowing. Now, all of her serves still weren't going over the net. She was missing balls. She tripped a time or two. But she could feel this shift deep within her: The moves weren't struggling out of her. They *were* her.

"My teacher looked so impressed," she said, "but also, kind of annoyed? Like he thought I had just not been trying before."

So that became Zuby's experience with embodiment. It was a shift from trying so hard your brain hurts to saying, "Fuck this, I have nothing to lose." Of course, in an ideal world, we would want that push to embodiment to come from a place of pure confidence and security, but sometimes having nothing to lose can give you that push you need to make a shift.

Zuby continued to use this experience to help her understand that being embodied would require nothing of her and everything of her at the same time. That it wouldn't come from being perfect or from an expert serve, but from a willingness to simply show up and take risks.

She began with just noticing when she felt performance anxiety and discovered she didn't just feel it in the sexual realm, but at work when she was speaking up at a meeting, or even in a busy restaurant when she felt pressure to decide and order quickly. After just observing for a while, Zuby began to let go of perfection and just adopt a "fuck this" attitude in lower stakes situations like the restaurant. Eventually she applied it to social and work situations, and ultimately a sexual scenario with her boyfriend.

A few weeks later she reported to me in my office, "I'd been noticing for a while the ways I wasn't in my body with Joel, especially when I started to worry I wasn't 'doing it right.' But I did what you recommended and waited till we weren't in the bedroom and just hanging out and told him the truth: that sometimes when we are intimate, I have trouble staying present because I'm worrying about whether I'm pleasing him or that I'm taking too long to please. He not only told me my concerns were ill founded . . ."

I grinned as Zuby playfully waggled her eyebrows with pride as she said this.

"But Joel also had a great idea! When I told him how I'd been trying what I'd named the 'fuck this strategy,' he suggested I start saying it out loud any time I notice I'm in my own head with insecurities. Then he'd know that I was feeling nervous and could reassure me, and I could remind myself to be with sex like tennis."

Just like with tennis, there were some awkward fumbles and trips at first. But eventually, with practice and Joel's encouragement and positive reinforcement, she began to fully enjoy sex magic and mind-blowing sex with Joel. And even when she inevitably still got in her own head sometimes, she had learned to ride the waves of insecurity or distraction with total faith that she'd easily find her balance once again.

CHAPTER 5

The Heart as a Path to Amazing Sex

> You have to love. You have to feel. It is the reason you are here on earth. You are here to risk your heart. You are here to be swallowed up.
>
> **—Louise Erdrich**

It has been said that your brain is the largest sex organ in your body. But did you know that the electromagnetic field your heart emits is sixty times greater than that of your brain? In fact, according to research from the Heartmath Institute, the electromagnetic field of the heart can be felt from up to thirty feet away. And your heart can actually synchronize with those you love. In a study published in *Infant Behavior and Development*, mothers and infants have been found to have synchronized heartbeats, even if they are separated by a few feet. And if the mother focuses on her baby and mentally channels her energy and thoughts to her baby, that synchronization becomes even more likely.

The same has been found for couples. Partners who share a bed have been found to have similar heartbeat patterns and breathing rhythms during the night. This also happens when they sit close to one another. And this connection doesn't happen with just anyone.

Researchers at the HeartMath Institute found that paired-up strangers do not synchronize with one another—it is just lovers who enjoy this bond and electromagnetic connection.

But what if you're single? Don't worry, your heart is still a powerful force. And you can use it as a lighthouse to call in the partner you desire. The knowledge that your heart will learn to entrain with—or tune into—your future partner in such a deep way can help you to make more conscious and enlightened dating choices. Because you now know that it's not just your body and your mind you're giving to your partner. You're literally sharing heart-space with them and giving them spiritual influence over your body's most crucial organ. When you think of love that way, you won't be as inclined to settle for second best. You won't let yourself be treated poorly by partners who aren't spiritually aligned with you.

THE POWER OF HEART-LED SEX

Heart-led sex doesn't have to mean sex that is slow or gentle. You can be as far from vanilla as you wish and still have heart-led sex.

Heart-led sex is about being willing to be at peace with all that is unhealed and unsolved inside of you, and all that is unhealed and unsolved inside of your partner. It also means that you are willing to show up open and vulnerable, rather than guarded and closed off to intimate connection.

But if you're like most people, when you think of adventurous, passionate sex, you don't think of fully committed, vulnerable, and secure partners who fully trust each other. You don't picture messy and authentic and imperfect people.

You might picture people from Hollywood rom-coms or from pornography. You might picture two strangers pulling each other's

THE HEART AS A PATH TO AMAZING SEX

clothes off in a bar bathroom. You might picture an unrequited love being fulfilled at long last when a person finally catches their crush's eye. You might picture a BDSM scenario occurring between a boss and his secretary, or a bodice-ripping fantasy straight from your favorite *Bridgerton* episode.

When I hear people talking about wanting adventure in the bedroom, I encourage them to really sit there and think about what they mean by that. You can buy all the lingerie and sex aids you want and try all the BDSM activities you desire, but if you're not taking emotional risks, all the external risks are just a meaningless show.

When they say they want adventure or spice, I ask my clients to go deeper and consider what they imagine the novelty will deliver. "Excitement" is what they usually say next, but that can mean many different things: nervous excitement, physical excitement, emotional excitement, and more. As we drill further and further down, we find that *intensity* is what they are truly seeking in sex. And that is what sex magic delivers, especially when experienced with an open heart.

Emotional risk-taking is the accelerant that will take your sex life and orgasms into the stratosphere of intensity and pleasure. Whether you are newly dating or you have been together for decades, true emotional risk-taking is probably the kinkiest and scariest thing you'll ever try in the bedroom. And like all great risks, it has the greatest payoff in the end.

STRATEGIES FOR EMOTIONAL RISK-TAKING

How do you become an emotional risk-taker in the bedroom? How do you strip away your defenses and learn to have sex that is vulnerable, raw, and liberating?

Let's start with the basics. These real-time actions can be implemented right now. Once you start playing with these steps, you will be ready to take things even deeper.

Date Sober

Don't automatically reach for your bottle of wine or your THC vape pen just because it's date night. I find that many couples tend to have date nights only on nights that they have mood-altering substances, such as Saturday nights or special occasions like concerts.

If your date night is the only time each week or each month that you get to be alone with your partner, consider whether alcohol or other substances will contribute to your connection or impede it.

Limit Distractions

Consider your date activities. Do you always go out at nighttime and hit the same old pubs or dinner spots? Do you go to movies, comedy shows, and so on? Try turning date night on its head by going on a day date in which you have no outside distractions or noise. Go on a gentle hike or picnic at a local park. Doing this is automatically going to create space for authenticity and connection.

Try a date with absolutely no technology (other than music). For instance, maybe you turn off your phones from 7 to 8 PM, or maybe say no screens before bed. These rules can be very hard to stick to, but here's the good news: The harder it is for you to put your screens away, the more beneficial this small choice will be for you and your relationship.

Our screens serve as a barrier between us and as a portal that takes us away from our partner into a totally different realm. This isn't a bad

THE HEART AS A PATH TO AMAZING SEX

thing, and technology itself isn't the enemy. But look for the ways in which you use technology to numb out or to escape your current mood. Do you find yourself reaching for your phone whenever you and your partner have a disagreement? Do you hop online when you feel yourself getting annoyed by something they're saying or doing?

We can't create vulnerability without being present, and no one can do this with a phone in their hands.

Get Curious

Get really curious about your partner's day and their inner life. Whenever you have the opportunity to have a conversation with each other, whether that's at dinner or when you're in the car together, ask yourself whether you're making the most of these moments. Do you find yourself complaining about a coworker or talking about your kid's grades or worrying about finances?

These conversations have a time and place, but if you want to start deepening your connection to your partner, you need to cultivate these moments and consciously start fostering the bounty you desire. I often encourage couples to individually journal about these topics and talk about them with each other. But you could even use them as topics of conversation to take your connection to a deeper level.

Probing Topics

You can create a deeper emotional connection with your partner by asking them deeper questions. Try out some of the following with your partner. I guarantee you will learn something new about them and grow even closer.

SEX MAGIC

* What is your favorite song and why?
* What is your greatest accomplishment?
* What person did you most admire in your childhood?
* What is your greatest regret?
* What person, living or dead, would you most like to have dinner with and why?
* What is the best gift you ever received?
* When do you first remember feeling rejected?
* What were you most frightened of as a child?
* What is the worst thing you ever did to a friend?
* What do you think happens to us after we die?
* What fictional character do you first remember relating to?
* Have you ever had a supernatural experience?
* If you could see one part of the future in a crystal ball, what would you most like to see or learn?
* Would you rather be ten years younger or $100,000 richer?
* What is the best compliment your partner ever gave you?
* Have you ever broken a promise? Why?
* What is the best vacation you ever went on?
* If you could go back in time, what would you tell your ten-year-old self?
* What era in time would you like to travel back to?

Check In with Four Heart-Centered Questions

You can get curious about your relationship as well. I always encourage couples to ask themselves and each other these four questions at least once or twice a year:

THE HEART AS A PATH TO AMAZING SEX

* What's one thing you think we currently do really well together?
* What aspect of life is currently feeling burdensome for you and how can we work together to make it less heavy?
* When do you feel the safest, the most seen, and the most heard? What's one thing you most need to hear from me?
* Is there something you want us to do more often together to feel closer or more connected?

You have the power to deepen your connection with your partner at a moment's notice. By switching off the phone, quieting your minds, making space, and getting curious about witnessing each other for who you really are, you're automatically entering a world of vulnerability.

THE SEXUAL ENERGY BETWEEN YOU

One of the most beautiful sex magical ways I've found of creating deep intimacy, connection, and pleasure through sex is by consciously circling and sharing the sexual energy between you. Tantric traditions support the idea that during a sexual encounter between a male and a female—or between two people in their masculine and feminine states—sexual energy is received through the heart of the feminine and shared with the masculine through the genitals. The masculine's energy is received through the genitals and shared with the feminine through the heart. It becomes an endless energetic loop that continues to build, creating more intense arousal and orgasms. It doesn't matter what your sexual orientation or gender identity is. In every successful sexual relationship between two people, one of you is more in your masculine, or yang, and one of you is more in your feminine, or yin.

Here are some ways you can work with this dynamic. Note that if you do not identify as male or female or identify as transgender, just focus on whether you (and your partner) are more in your feminine (yin) or masculine (yang) energy during the sexual encounter and practice accordingly. For instance, let's suppose that anatomically you have a penis, but you identify as female (or enjoy being in your feminine during sex), and you are having sex with someone who identifies as male (or is in their masculine during sex). You would follow the instructions for the feminine having sex with the masculine and practice accordingly.

For the Feminine Who Is Having Sex with the Masculine

While being intimate, envision gorgeous, loving sexual energy and light flowing from your partner's heart into yours. Imagine the light of that energy flowing down through your chakras with your breath and building in intensity. Let it flow and pool in your genitals. Then as you breathe out, imagine the light flowing straight out your genitals and into your partner's genitals. Imagine a loop of energy between you, coming in through your partner's heart and flowing out through your genitals into theirs.

For the Masculine Who Is Having Sex with the Feminine

While being intimate, imagine receiving flowing light energy from your partner's genitals into yours, flowing through your root and sacral chakras and shooting up, all the way up to your heart chakra. Let it pool and build there for several breaths. On an out-breath, send the energy out of your heart and into your partner's heart. Imagine a loop of energy between you, coming in through your partner's genitals and flowing up and out through your heart into your partner's heart.

THE HEART AS A PATH TO AMAZING SEX

For Those Who Identify as Both Masculine and Feminine or Neither

You can experiment with what feels best. Circle the energy back and forth between your genitals, or back and forth between your hearts. This will create much more emotional as well as physical intensity. You can also try taking turns being the heart starter or genital starter, unless one of you enjoys one direction more than the other.

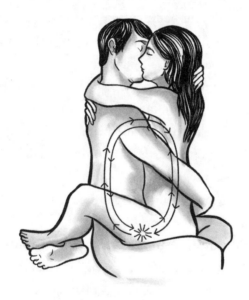

Couple in Yab Yum position circling energy

Soft Synchronized Gazing Breath

Soft synchronized gazing breath is also a beautiful way of deepening and intensifying intimacy and pleasure between you and your partner. It's a combination of synchronized breathing with something called "soft vision." With soft vision, we reverse the usual way we see one another. Instead of experiencing ourselves as looking outward, we focus on experiencing and imagining ourselves as receiving what we are gazing at inwardly through the eyes rather than looking out from them. On the quantum level this is already the case; there is no separation between us and anything else anatomically speaking. Through our soft gaze we are taking our partner into our selves through our vision. It starts by practicing soft vision on your own and then trying it with your partner.

1. Sit or lie comfortably and close your eyes to start, bringing awareness to your body, putting your attention on your heart center or your belly, whatever place can anchor you in awareness in the body.

2. Take some grounding breaths in through your nose and out through your mouth, imagining light flowing in through the top of your head with the in-breath, and flowing out your tail bone deep into the earth with the out-breath, grounding you in the present moment.

3. Very slowly open your eyes, millimeter by millimeter, allowing whatever your increasing gaze takes in to fall *into you* through your eyes. Imagine taking what you see into your body and your being. Simply imagine whatever is before you, which your eyes are taking in, actually entering you. Stay connected to your body and what you are feeling there. It's okay if you notice you have left your body awareness. Close your eyes and reconnect inwardly for several breaths, then slowly and gently open your eyes again.

4. Once you feel comfortable soft gazing around the room, it's time to try soft gazing at your partner. It works the same way, but in this case, you are taking your partner's being into you through your eyes.

THE HEART AS A PATH TO AMAZING SEX

5. Now it's time to add in simultaneous breathing, which takes the intensity to the next level. Both you and your partner breathe in and out at the same time and rate, synchronized. The breaths should be deep and slow, sending the air toward the belly and the genitals with your awareness or visualization. Breathe in for the count of four and out for the count of six. If you slip out of rhythm, no worries; just relax for a few breaths and sync back up together.

PRESENCE AND VULNERABILITY IN THE BEDROOM AND BEYOND

Now, how can you take things even deeper? How can you cultivate this kind of conscious rawness in the bedroom?

Begin by asking yourself how it would feel *in your body* if you were bared, body and soul, before your partner. How would it feel physically if you had no secrets from your partner? No tricks, no shadows, no games, no hiding places.

Be willing to sit with the feelings that come up and let any discomfort just happen. Name what is happening to your partner so they don't feel just a brick wall of energy coming from you. Say something like, "I am feeling triggered today and I'm not sure why. It's making me not want to talk, but I want you to know I love you so much and it's not your fault. I am just hurting right now," or "I know I'm being extra clingy and talkative today. I think I'm feeling really lonely and scared, and I'm not sure where those feelings are coming from."

Be willing to give your partner the same patience and understanding when they are exhibiting behavior that you might not fully understand. Resist the urge to write yourself as the main character in their emotional world. Whether your partner is quiet and shut down or more jealous and snappier than normal, consciously refuse to make up any stories about what might be going on. Picture a protective bubble around you that will help you maintain your own energy, and channel that peace and calm toward them.

You don't have to be a doormat or accept negative treatment from your partner (or anyone), but begin playing with the idea that your partner's mood is not your fault, nor your responsibility. You cannot tend to their emotional self-regulation as well as your own. It is amazing how much faster your partner will move through a bad mood or a period of sadness if you are willing to sit with them rather than challenge them or question them, and especially if you are willing to hold your own emotional center rather than jump into their storm.

How can you apply this kind of presence and acceptance into better orgasms and more meaningful and passionate sex?

First, understand that all these actions you are taking outside of the bedroom are going to pay off inside the bedroom as well. If your partner feels more seen and held by you, they're going to feel safer being more vulnerable during sex, even if they don't quite know why or realize what is happening. The same will be true for you.

Second, start looking for the ways in which you hide sexually. Maybe you close your eyes frequently during physical intimacy, or you don't like your partner to see your face. Maybe you fake orgasm or pretend something feels good when it doesn't. Maybe you don't try the positions you really want to try because you're scared your partner won't like it. You might be afraid of seeming afraid, of seeming shy or awkward. You might revert to bravado with lots of dirty talk or other distractions because you want to make it seem like you're totally confident.

Do you find that you're often reverting to little parlor tricks to keep your partner from really seeing you? Or from noticing that you're

THE HEART AS A PATH TO AMAZING SEX

not a perfect sexual god/goddess, but that you're a flawed person with cellulite, scars, sexual shame, and baggage? What would happen if you took that fantasy off the table and confessed to your partner, "Sometimes during sex, I feel really incompetent or like I'm not good enough," or "When we make love, I am scared to try new stuff and look silly."

I bet if you told your partner this, they would say, "Me too!" Once we stop trying to act so cool in the bedroom and start making space for our real, messy, uncool selves, we find out the very cool fact that *no one* feels invulnerable in the bedroom. We might hide and pretend and put on shows for each other, but deep down, we're all wanting to be desired and loved, and we're all fearing that we won't be and that we maybe don't even deserve to be.

Stripping away these falsehoods and letting the truth out can be so freeing. It's also the path to fully experiencing sex magic. The more you release the distractions of inhibitions and insecurities, the more present you can be in your body, in the experience, and with your partner.

Not to mention, when you confess these truths, you make room for your partner to do the same. "I like giving you oral, but it makes me feel awkward because I don't think I'm that good at it," or "I want to break out of our usual routine but I don't think I'm sexy enough or brave enough to just go for it."

You foster an environment in which no one has to play a part or fake it till they make it. This creates the kind of safety and security that will allow you to take risks and try new things sexually. It creates conversations that will be tender, funny, and meaningful.

You have the power to stand in your relationship as a vulnerable, brave partner. You can rewrite the status quo of your sex life.

143

RELATIONSHIP IMPLICATIONS FOR THE EMPATH

Are you an empath? Empaths are deeply feeling people who are intensely connected to their hearts and the hearts of others. They not only feel their own emotions but the emotions of other people around them as well. Empaths often take on these emotions as their own, experiencing the grief, fear, anger, and joy of other people, even if these people are strangers to them.

While empaths can feel the emotions of anyone in their world, even fictional characters in books and movies, they will feel most deeply the emotions of their loved ones. The emotional lives of the people closest to them will impact them on such a personal level that they might not be able to differentiate between their own emotions and the emotions of their loved ones.

Empaths definitely have superpowers, but the risk is for the kind of empath who can't be okay if the people they love aren't. If their partner is having a bad day, they're having a bad day. If their best friend is heartbroken, they're heartbroken. If their child is stressed out, they're stressed out. If their dog is sick, they almost feel sick themselves.

As a therapist, an empath, and a recovering codependent, I can tell you that empaths are almost always also codependent. It's the way we learned to survive our childhoods. We not only needed to sense what was happening in the caretakers in charge in order to stay safe, but we were praised and approved of when we pushed our own needs off to the side and attended to everyone else's needs instead.

Ask yourself this: When you are feeling the emotions of everyone around you, are you connecting with them, or are you trying to control them? Are you still fully in your own body, or have you left it and begun embodying their experience instead?

THE HEART AS A PATH TO AMAZING SEX

We must recognize that lighting ourselves on fire to keep other people warm isn't a selfless act. It's a fearful act, an act of isolation and self-abandonment instead of connection. Instead, when you see yourself going into intense people-pleasing mode, stop and ask yourself what need you are trying to meet inside of yourself. You'll often find that you're avoiding something that might feel challenging or uncomfortable.

SEXUAL IMPLICATIONS FOR EMPATHS

If you or your partner are an empath, it will impact your sexual connection. One common issue for empaths is that they struggle to experience what is happening inside their own body because they are so busy experiencing what is happening inside other people's bodies. You can imagine how this will play out during intimacy. An empath will often be so wrapped up in ensuring that their partner is enjoying as much pleasure as possible that they are subconsciously preventing themselves from enjoying pleasure. They aren't present in their own bodies. Ironically, this will negatively impact their partner's pleasure as well.

The best gift you can give your partner is your full attention and presence in the bedroom, and that includes inhabiting yourself. Empaths don't often realize this, but we can use our empathy as a barrier against vulnerability. When we live others' emotions, we don't have to live our own, and we don't have to display them or allow them to potentially be judged.

In a sexual scenario, this can look like someone who is almost exclusively a "giver," more concerned with pleasuring their partner than receiving pleasure themselves. While giving is important for great sex, receiving is just as important. And learning to be a receiver can be much more difficult than learning to be a giver, especially for empaths.

To receive you must believe that you are worthy of the gifts being offered to you. To receive you must be willing and desirous of being cherished. That can be a very tough ask, and it can bring lots of painful emotions that you might have been avoiding without even realizing it.

When you think about a night in which your partner worships your body, what do you feel inside? Shy, awkward, and maybe even resistant? Does the thought of being adored by your partner while you actively do nothing except receive that adoration make you feel unworthy or even ashamed?

Now, try to connect to how that would feel physically. Visualize how you would feel physically if your partner was catering to your sexual needs and worshiping your body. Where would you feel those physical sensations? Would you be able to feel it in your genitals? Would you feel warmth or tingling across your body?

Or maybe you would feel nothing at all. When you slow down and pay attention to the physical sensations you experience during sex, you might be surprised to discover that you're not feeling very much of anything.

This is because you have literally trained your body not to have needs and not to experience any sensations. Like an ignored hunger cue, your brain learns to dismiss sensations that won't receive attention. So, when you finally return to your body after so many years of having self-less sex, you might be shocked to find that your body has kept the score. It has been trained to turn itself off, to make itself small and unimportant. This is the bitter cost an empath can pay.

But don't worry. You can build that neural connection once again. It will take time and conscious effort to bring yourself back into the bedroom. You will have to learn to receive. You will have to learn to let yourself be worthy.

THE HEART AS A PATH TO AMAZING SEX

SEXUAL WORTHINESS FOR WOMEN

Researchers have found that a person's confidence in their ability to accomplish necessary tasks—or self-efficacy—plays a large role in women's ability to enjoy sexual pleasure. The study, which was published in the journal *Archives of Sexual Behavior*, found that women with higher sexual self-esteem, higher self-efficacy, and higher belief in their entitlement to sexual pleasure had more frequent orgasms than women who rated lower in these categories.

This survey is very important because it shows that improving sexual pleasure for women comes down to more than just foreplay, better techniques, and circumventing common female sexual function issues. Of course, those things are important, and I cover them in many of my other books. But the truth is, all the lingerie and date nights in the world won't mean a thing if the woman wearing the fishnet bodysuit doesn't feel like she's truly worthy of sexual pleasure and truly capable of creating it.

So do you really feel like you are deserving of sexual pleasure? Do you view yourself as a sexy and desirable being who can create orgasms for herself and her partner? If the answer is no, that's okay. Acknowledge that reality—but add a *yet*. For example, "I am not confident in the bedroom—yet," or "I don't fully own my sexual side—yet." Make space for the possibility that this can change in the future, and then take steps to make that happen. That might mean journaling, meditation, therapy, or self-exploration. It might mean making a promise to yourself to stop faking orgasm. It might mean making time every week for masturbation. Just make a commitment to honor those feelings of insecurity rather than running away from them, or assuming it doesn't matter if you don't feel confident in the bedroom. It does matter, greatly—to you, to your partner, and to your growth here on this planet. If you want more ideas for building authentic sexual entitlement, you can also check out my book *Real Sex for Real Women*.

SEXUAL WORTHINESS FOR MEN

You are not required to "perform" in the bedroom. It's common to hear the phrase "sexual performance" and it's almost always referring to the male partner: how long they can last, how well they can make love, and how skilled they are in making their partner achieve orgasms.

If you are a male empath, this will exponentially increase your stress in the bedroom. Not only will your unique emotional makeup cause you to focus more on how your partner is feeling than how *you* are feeling, but you have years of social conditioning telling you how men "should" behave in the bedroom, such as that men "should":

* Always be in the mood for sex
* Always be ready to go, meaning that they should achieve an erection and be ready to "perform" at a moment's notice
* Be able to have meaningless sex with many partners
* Be virile, tough, and not feel emotional about sex
* Know how to pleasure a woman without needing her input or advice

No wonder men can find lovemaking so stressful. They're being asked to perform like a circus animal rather than show up as a whole, vulnerable human being. They have to adopt a certain machismo about sex and pretend like they are always in the mood and that things like stress and anxiety never dampen their libido. And they can never admit that sometimes they really, really just want to snuggle, and maybe even to be the little spoon.

So if you're a man reading this, I want you to know: It's not your duty to deliver orgasms to your partner on a silver platter. Orgasms are something you make together. Sex is an act of connection, not a performance. The best kind of sex is the sex we have when we aren't playing a part, when we aren't trying to live up to ridiculous standards created by faceless strangers.

SEX MAGIC CASE FILE

When I first met Norah, I was instantly taken with her charm and warmth, which seemed to envelop the room in a bright light. She seemed like someone who had it all. She was a college professor at a top state college, and she had two healthy kids and a supportive and loving partner of twenty years.

At first, it was hard to find out what was *really* going on inside Norah's mind. She chattered a mile a minute, with great humor and intelligence. I quietly let her have the floor for a while, internally noticing how hard she was working to make me like her. There was a quiet desperation there that was hidden behind her chic haircut and her impeccable appearance.

Finally, Norah dropped her mask for a moment and confessed that her marriage was on the rocks.

"We haven't had sex in three years," she said. "I can't believe I am even admitting that."

It wasn't that she didn't love Paul. The pair did almost everything together. They walked to work side by side every morning and spent their weekends with their kids, the four of them always together and enjoying parties, friends, sports, and other adventures.

So what was wrong? Why had they stopped having sex?

At first, Norah pointed to common issues that many parents and busy people have. Not enough time. Not enough sleep. Too much stress. Not enough alone time. Too much time on the go and not enough time in the present.

Except Norah was massively intelligent. She consumed lots of media about relationships and intimacy. She devoured books and podcasts about having a better sex life. She had implemented the date nights and vacations away without the kids. She had the lingerie and the sex toys and the babysitter on speed dial.

Over a few sessions of working together, I came to realize that underneath this cool and calm façade was a very angry and very hurt woman. She had a breezy, lighthearted exterior that belied the rock of emotions within her.

This anger came out in small stories. The frustration with how her daughter forgot her schoolbook at home that morning. The rage that Paul was fifteen minutes late to their eldest's softball game that weekend. The irritation that her work wasn't being as celebrated in her department as she hoped.

Simply put, Norah was so, so hard on herself and everyone she loved. She wanted perfection like she wanted air to breathe. But in order to be liked, she oozed charm and warmth even as she quietly seethed and fell apart in private every time something went wrong in her life.

She was trying to be needless and unproblematic, easily liked and easily admired. She didn't want to be a work in progress, an imperfect and flawed human—because she didn't believe anyone could love someone like that.

"You mentioned that Penny left her schoolbook at home this morning," I said. "Can you tell me a time when you did something similar in your childhood? How did your parents react?"

THE HEART AS A PATH TO AMAZING SEX

Norah let out a sharp laugh.

"My parents would have killed me," she said. "Forgetting things, being a few minutes late, getting in trouble at school . . . that was grounds for punishment."

"What did punishment look like for little you?"

Norah explained that being grounded meant that she had to come right home from school and sit in her room. No phone or television or music. She could do her homework, but once that was done, she could do nothing but sit on her bed (sit, not lie) until bedtime. Dinner was brought to her on a tray by her silent and disapproving parents. Then, it was time to brush teeth and go to bed. These punishments could last for days or weeks. Once over, it was never discussed.

So for the crime of childlike mistakes, such as forgetting a schoolbook, walking too slowly to the bus stop, or talking during class, Norah was punished with extreme isolation. And after that rupture, there was no repair. There was no hugging and discussion. It was just business as usual, until Norah made another mistake and was punished once again.

"Being alone like that must have been brutal for you," I said. "You're such a social spirit."

"Yes," she agreed. "It was never as hard on my older sister. She is good at being alone. She would tell herself stories and imagine things. I couldn't do that. I was too miserable. I was just so ashamed."

"Ashamed to be punished that way?" I asked.

"No," said Norah. "Ashamed to have made a mistake in the first place. See, my sister resents my parents for those days, but I know they made me stronger. It wasn't like they abused us. They just wanted us to be better."

"To be better so they could love you."

Norah nodded, then paused. "No, wait . . . I mean they always loved us."

151

She looked uncomfortable.

"They might have said 'I love you' before bed every night, but what I am hearing is that you weren't given love, which for kids is approval, unless you were perfect," I said. "In fact, the slightest mistake would lead to rejection with no repair; in the form of isolation and devastating aloneness that broke little Norah's spirit. That little girl learned that the only way to be safe from that kind of abandonment was to be perfect."

And now, at the age of forty-three, adult Norah was still carrying those wounds. The desire to be perfect and to make that perfection appear effortless was her main concern every day. This was an issue for her throughout her dating life. Before she met Paul, she would routinely date men who used her almost as a mother figure. She helped her college boyfriend pass his classes, she helped her next boyfriend start up his new business, and she helped the next one get out of debt and stop drinking.

Everywhere she went, she was a fixer. And as she described her sexual experiences, I realized this was true in the bedroom too. She had often faked orgasms in the past with Paul, and she didn't let him perform oral sex on her. She hated her body and didn't like having sex in the shower or with the lights on.

"Maybe when I lose ten pounds," she said. "That's what I keep telling myself. That we will start having sex again once I lose weight. Or when I have more time to go to the gym. When the kids are older or are better at managing their own schoolwork . . ."

It was always some distant "when" that never came, because Norah was waiting for a time when she was perfect. "I want you to learn how to be okay even when you're a mess," I said. "I want you to feel deserving of love and pleasure even on your most broken days."

THE HEART AS A PATH TO AMAZING SEX

Together, Norah and I began a low-stakes way for her to start experimenting with not being perfect. She began by not cleaning the house when her in-laws came over for a visit. (She told me that she would usually stay up until 3 AM scrubbing and polishing every inch of her home for guests.)

Letting go of some of her perfectionism wasn't easy for Norah, but she learned how to handle that part of herself gently. We did Somatic Experiencing to help move some of the locked trauma she had from her childhood. We worked on scripts to help her respond to criticisms from her own parents, which was a big point of pain and contention for her because they would often degrade her or her accomplishments in a joking manner. No wonder Norah learned to have a cool and unflappable exterior.

And finally, we got to the root of why her attraction to Paul waned in the first place. As a Type A perfectionist who wanted everything to be "just so," she often took on the role of bossing Paul around (although not intentionally). And, as a natural people-pleaser with a gentler and more passive personality, Paul took the role of her employee quite naturally. But unfortunately this dynamic did a number on their sex life. Norah had to learn how to be okay with imperfections—a messy house, a missed soccer game, a hasty birthday party without Pinterest-worthy decor. She had to learn that her sex life and her connection with Paul was more important than micromanaging the way he loaded the dishwasher or the way he cut the lawn. Not only did her attraction to Paul increase when she started viewing him as more of a partner and less of a child to be bossed around, but his attraction to her increased when he was able to see her as a sexy, vibrant woman rather than the person who was going to scold him for being late to a dance recital.

As with Norah, your sexual self-worth might be connected to so many different pieces of your history. It might be tied to the way your parents treated you when you made mistakes. It might be tied to the way you feel about being seen and being vulnerable. It might be tied to the way you feel toward your partner when they make mistakes and when they are vulnerable. Be curious. Be willing to investigate. Play with possible solutions and potential approaches.

CHAPTER 6

Cultivating Sexual Power

> Force is pompous; it has all the answers. Power is unassuming. Force needs to control others because it lacks power, just as vanity stems from a lack of self-esteem.
>
> **—David Hawkins**

Sex magic requires you to stand in your sexual power. To create sex magic you must realize how sexually powerful you are and how immensely sexually capable you are. You must be willing to step into that power.

Sexual power might not sound desirable, especially if you identify as a highly "feminine" person. Sexual power sounds to some like a state that is forceful and even aggressive. It might sound like someone who takes charge and doesn't take no for an answer.

But that notion misunderstands the true meaning of power. Power and force have nothing to do with one another. In fact, they are opposites in many ways.

How so?

When you *force* someone to do something, they lose their agency. They lose their self-respect as well as their respect for you. They're operating out of a place of fear.

When you are in your power, you don't compel—you lead. You influence. You manifest. You create.

You know the difference between power and force almost immediately. When someone barks an order at you, it makes you feel small. You might feel foolish or embarrassed. Why do you feel that way? Because you are responding to the energy of that forceful individual, and you can feel the control, or even anger. Despite how it may appear, that person also feels small and foolish. They're grappling with low self-worth and trying to exert control and dominion over what's happening in their world. They're terrified of mistakes and of not being perfect. They fear judgment more than anything, and they are desperate to avoid criticism and vulnerability.

Now compare that to a person who, instead of giving an order, makes a firm request from a place of power. They're not afraid of criticism. They're not afraid to take big risks and make big mistakes. They believe they live in a universe that is kind, supportive, and has their back. They believe in their inherent self-worth and dignity, and they believe in yours as well.

So when they give you tasks, you respond to that energy of groundedness. You feel capable. You feel protected. You feel powerful too. This means you can make mistakes, ask questions, take risks, and be your whole, vulnerable self.

Now put that scenario into a sexual experience. A person who is sexually forceful is a person who probably feels very weak and even unlovable at their core. They don't believe any partner would willingly desire them, at least not if they had other options. They don't feel as equal to the people around them, especially not the people they see as sexually desirable.

Sexual force doesn't have to mean forcing other people to engage in sex acts. It could mean forcing yourself to submit to sex that doesn't feel good. It could mean forcing yourself to fake orgasms or have multiple partners or otherwise engage in sexual activities that don't ultimately serve your goals. It could mean forcing yourself to stay invulnerable and unreachable during sex, to put barriers around your heart so you don't get hurt.

Let's compare that to someone who is sexually powerful. They feel safe and secure in their bodies, in their desires, and in their capabilities. Having sex with someone who is sexually powerful makes you feel that same way. They feel grounded and centered and in control of themselves. As a result, you can feel freer to be vulnerable, to try new things, and to simply exist as your whole self.

Simply put, power makes you feel good. It makes the people around you feel good. It turns you from a victim into a hero in your own story. And this gives you the ability to direct how you want your story to go. You don't have to wait for your partner to "give" you orgasms. You don't have to lose twenty pounds before you get to feel sexy. You don't have to be afraid to ask for what you want or to say when something isn't working for you.

When we are powerful, we are inhabiting ourselves. And we hold space for our partners to do the same.

UNDERSTANDING WHAT *ISN'T* SEXUAL POWER

When you think of sexual power, I don't want you to envision handcuffs or other BDSM acts. Not that BDSM isn't perfectly healthy and okay to enjoy, and you can stand in your sexual power and enjoy BDSM. But many people can get distracted by the bells and whistles of sexual games and not realize that they have left their sexual power at the door.

Let's examine common ways that people use force in the bedroom and ways that they would be better served by using their sexual power:

Sex as a Manipulation Tactic

Carey has been hooking up with her friend Frank for over a year. They met at work, and she instantly fell for him. He liked her as well, and they often flirted and spent time together outside of work. But Frank was a player who made it clear that he didn't "do monogamy." Carey was heartbroken by this but pretended not to be. Instead, she let things progress and told him she would be fine with "no-strings-attached sex."

This continued for months. She kept having sex with him in the hope that he would see she was the one for him. He enjoyed their time together but was continuing to see other women as promised. She began to feel desperate and started to be even kinkier and wilder during sex. She tried to appear as though she didn't have needs so that he would see she wouldn't be a stereotypical nagging girlfriend. So she acted like she didn't care that he never took her on dates or that he forgot her birthday.

Finally, in a last-ditch attempt to get his attention, she started hooking up with other partners as well. She found random men to flirt with, preferably in front of Frank. She drank more often and stopped taking care of her body, at least on the inside. On the outside, she was working out, skipping carbs, and spending most of her paycheck

CULTIVATING SEXUAL POWER

on makeup, clothes, lingerie—anything to get Frank's attention. He dominated her thoughts and her conversations, to the point that her friends would internally cringe when she mentioned his name.

This is an all-too-typical scenario that I have seen many times with my clients. People try to use sex to keep or catch a partner, only to wind up feeling used themselves. They try to manipulate or fool their partner into falling for this false, perfect version of themselves, but in the end they are the ones who wind up feeling manipulated.

Now, what would have happened if Carey used power rather than force? How would things have worked out differently?

She would still have met Frank and flirted with him. They would still have had that instant attraction and excitement around each other. But when he made it clear that he didn't want a monogamous relationship, she would have paused. She would know that hooking up wasn't what she wanted. So she would pull back from Frank and stop wasting her energy on a relationship that was going nowhere.

Maybe Frank would have eventually realized that Carey really was the one and he was ready to settle down. But maybe he wouldn't have. So in both scenarios, it's totally possible that Carey and Frank wouldn't wind up together and she wouldn't get her happily ever after with him.

But in the latter scenario, she wouldn't have wasted two of her most precious commodities—time and energy—on a painful, dead-end relationship. She could have used that time to focus on her own needs and goals, and she would be open to finding Mr. Right instead of being completely distracted by her non-relationship with Frank. She wouldn't have to use shopping or substances to numb her pain, and instead could have practiced self-care and spent time on her hobbies, career, and friendships.

The Carey in that scenario is so powerful. She's sexy. She's capable. She loves herself and she consciously tries to build a beautiful life for herself.

And the only difference is that she moved from a place of force (a place of ego, fear, and unworthiness) and into a place of power (a place of hope, faith, and self-love).

Sex as a Self-Soothing Tactic

A sexually powerful person can grapple with feelings of discomfort. They can endure and even learn from the reality that no one is young and beautiful forever. They can work through the grief of lost loves and sit with the uncertainty of what comes next. They can be honest about their sexual needs and sexual motivations. And, most important, they can soothe themselves with something other than sex.

Here is the most important thing to know about sexual power: When you are in your sexual power, you know that sex is about connection, not competition. You don't use sex as a tool for manipulation, but as a tool for healing and pleasure. You honor your body and your sexuality, and you do the same for your partner.

Sex as a Form of Revenge

Revenge sex can be sneaky. Sometimes it can look like healing. Sometimes it can look like "moving on."

For example, after a painful breakup, many people want to find another partner quickly, even if it's just for a one-night stand. This is especially true if your ex has moved on or maybe even betrayed you during your relationship. Seeing your ex with a new partner might trigger you into seeking attention and affection from someone else.

CULTIVATING SEXUAL POWER

I've even seen many people have revenge sex after deciding to stay with a partner who cheated, in a misguided attempt to "even the playing field."

The problem with revenge sex is that you are abandoning your sexual power when you partake in it. You are letting someone else dictate your most intimate choices. Standing in your sexual power, you are able to feel the pain of feeling unwanted, mistreated, or abandoned, while understanding this doesn't have to be your future and you can and will be loved, held, and cherished again.

Simply put, sexual power sometimes looks like *not* having sex. But don't look at it as a dry spell. In fact, this can be a very fertile time for you. This can be a time when you plant deep seeds, prune unwanted branches, and tend to your growth. It can be a time when you are utterly self-concerned. And you can still enjoy erotica, self-stimulation, and fantasy.

You will know when the time is right. You will know because the feeling will come not out of desperation or loneliness. It will come when you have a full cup. It will come when you already feel safe, seen, and valued. Sex cannot give you these things. Only you can. And then you will know true sexual power.

Sex Without Boundaries

When is the last time you said no in the bedroom? When you have boundaries, the word "no" isn't loaded with implications. You can say no and still be loved. You can say no and still be safe in your relationship. It doesn't mean you aren't attracted to each other. It doesn't mean that there is something wrong with either of you.

Remember that practice makes perfect when it comes to boundaries. Say no to people until it feels like second nature. Start by saying no in low-stakes ways, such as to participating in a neighborhood block party or buying cookies for a fundraiser. You can also practice boundaries just by expressing your honest opinion when you might normally go with the flow. Maybe you don't like the latest hit television show, a certain artist, or a brand of clothing. Practice expressing a contrary opinion about minor things and feel that tension and fear in your belly. Notice that it is really hard for you. And let that discomfort be okay.

Soon you can move on to saying no to other, higher stakes things, like the project at work that you really don't want to take on, or the friend who always calls late at night when you're about to go to bed, or the expectation of hosting the entire family for the holidays.

The more you can practice this skill outside the bedroom, the more you can implement it in the bedroom. Remember, "no" is not a moral judgment. It's not an insult or an attack. It's a safe word. It's a word that keeps love safe and keeps sex safe.

Sex as a Band-Aid

Couples can use sex to avoid other issues in their relationships. Some people have regular sex but haven't kissed their partner in months. Others enjoy active sex lives but haven't had a real conversation with their partner in years.

Sex should equal intimacy, but it often doesn't. It's easy to have un-intimate sex if you are used to it. It's easy to go on date night and have a few glasses of wine, then come home and have completely disconnected sex.

It's a way to pretend that everything is okay—a way to avoid looking at the places in your life that aren't working, the places in your relationship that need tending. Sex can be used as a temporary

Band-Aid the same way we might use a cup of hot tea or a candy bar as a pick-me-up after a bad day. But ideally we don't approach sex the way we approach the Starbucks drive-thru, as a fast, thoughtless way to boost our dopamine.

Don't get me wrong: Maintenance sex can be used to keep intimacy alive, and there is nothing wrong with "quickies." But when we are just going through the motions and performing sex almost in a rote, thoughtless way, we aren't in our power. If you aren't present and fully engaged, you're not fully empowered. If your mind is on your to-do list or the fact that you missed the gym too much this month, you're not owning your sexual self-worth and you're not able to fully connect to your partner. So just be aware of your mindset even when you're having maintenance sex.

OWNING DIVINE FEMININE *AND* MASCULINE SEXUAL POWER

Although we are all energy, our energies are completely unique. In Chinese philosophy, the terms "yin" and "yang" are used to describe the two distinct types of energy that were born out of the chaos of nothingness.

Yin and yang are the two forces that shaped and formed all creation. Dark and light. Fire and water. Man and woman. Night and day. Young and old. Positive and negative. North and south. East and west. Birth and death. Above and below.

Yin and yang are the unity of opposites. One cannot exist without the other. Without darkness, there would be no such thing as light. Without birth, there would be no such thing as death. Without the feminine, there would be no such thing as the masculine. When we own both the masculine and feminine within us and let the balance of the two express in the most authentic of ways, we can truly be in our full sexual power.

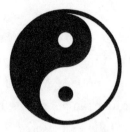

The yin and yang symbol

The symbol of yin and yang (陰陽 / 阴阳 in Chinese characters) is made of two half circles, one white and one black, each with a small dot of the opposite shade in its center. Because although these forces may seem opposing, they are inherently united. These forces are constantly fueling and influencing one another. Without end, throughout time, these unified opposites are responsible for creating and sustaining everything we experience in this universe.

Similarly, each of us has yin and yang energy. Yin is the feminine energy. It is restive, emotional, open, fluid, cool, intuitive, and oriented inward. Yin is soft, receptive, and deep. In nature, yin is represented by the Moon, darkness, water, and the seasons autumn and winter. You might expect yin to be spring or summer, because feminine energy is often associated with new life and things like blossoms, buds, and warmth.

But yin energy is inward. It is *receiving*. It's the deep well of emotional, spiritual, and creative expression. During autumn and winter, life is still being created. The new life that we see around us in spring is not just the result of brighter, warmer days; it is the result of the darkness, the coolness, the decomposition, the restive forces of creation that were happening under the surface of the Earth during the cooler months. Are you starting to see the delicate dance between the opposing forces that author and nourish all life on this Earth?

In nature, yang is the earth. It is fire, it is heat, it is active and directive. If yin is the flowing cool river of rolling waters, yang is the riverbank, containing and directing. While the creative powers of yin are restive, yang is active. It is external. Yang is spring and summer, yang is life exploding all over the place under the bright, fierce rays of the Sun. Yang is movement. Yang is action. Yang's power is loud, aggressive, and external.

In the bedroom, we all have yin and yang energy. There is some real truth to the idea of "opposites attract," especially when it comes to masculine and feminine energy, yin and yang. In relationships, it's the polarity between the masculine and the feminine that creates chemistry. Remember, I am not talking about gender, but energy. An individual identifying as a man and/or with male sexual anatomy can be more in his feminine energy and vice versa. The greater the polarity between the masculine and feminine, the stronger the attraction, intimate connection, and sexual energies between two people are.

In addition to having a polarity in the yin and yang energy balance between you, it is crucial to be in alignment and balanced in the yin and yang energy *within* you. Connecting to and understanding that energy is so important, because they can easily get out of balance. An overactive yang or an overactive yin can lead to disconnection and disruption in the body, as can an underactive yang or an underactive yin.

What does an overactive yang look like? Someone who is very externally focused in the bedroom. An overactive yang can lead you to behave selfishly, impulsively, or aggressively. You won't be able to slow down, be in the moment, or get deeper than just your physical sensations.

An overactive yin can lead to someone who is very passive, inhibited, or trapped in their mind. If your yin is overactive, you might struggle to express your needs or connect to your physical sensations. An overactive yin can even lead you to disassociate from your body and be too much in your own head. And, since you and your partner are deeply connected, if your yin or yang are overactive, it can trigger their energy to go too far into yin or yang territory as well.

The goal is to find harmony between yin and yang. Your yin-yang harmony will be unique to you, and it may change over time. There may be times when you are more connected to yin energy in the bedroom, and that doesn't mean that you aren't in harmony with yang. But if you have *no* yang energy or you are really working hard to suppress your yang energy, that is going to throw a wrench in your ability to create sexual pleasure for your partner and you.

What can cause our yin or yang to get out of whack?

Your sexual energy is deeply informed by the culture, religion, and family you grew up in. It is also deeply informed by your early sexual experiences, including the media you consumed and the way your friends and social group talked about sex. And, of course, it will be deeply informed by things like childhood sexual trauma, your first sexual partners, and how comfortable you felt expressing your sexual orientation or your gender identity.

A woman who received a lot of negative messages about female sexuality and how "nice girls" don't enjoy sex or want a lot of sex might have very overactive yin energy. This will present as being very inhibited in the bedroom. They might be afraid to be vocal or take charge of their sexual pleasure. They will be completely passive in the bedroom and unwilling to initiate or own their sexual power.

Someone who experienced sexual trauma as a child might have overactive yin or they might also have overactive yang. People with

CULTIVATING SEXUAL POWER

childhood sexual trauma can learn to approach sexual pleasure without any emotional connection, to shut down their spiritual self entirely in the bedroom. They might use sex addictively, such as compulsively watching pornography, cheating on their partners, or being self-destructively promiscuous.

One of the best ways to improve your sexual pleasure and help you step into your creative sexual power is by getting in touch with your yin and yang energy and ensuring that you aren't suppressing or limiting your whole sexual self.

GAINING ACCESS TO YOUR YIN AND YANG ENERGIES

Get your testes breathing, your vagina sparkling, and your bottom moving!

Let's look at three different exercises to access both yin and yang energies: one for people with penises, one for those with vaginas, and one for anyone with a bottom! These techniques maximize energy and sensation in your genital region for you as well as your partner, either during the exercise itself or as a result of learning to cultivate these techniques.

Testicular Breathing

Here's one especially for the guys. Testicular breathing is a great exercise for men who want to extend their staying power and as a way to move and build sexual energy.

1. Sit on a chair with your back straight but relaxed. Distribute your weight to your buttocks and feet. You do not want your genitals to be in contact with the chair itself.

167

SEX MAGIC

2. Bring your attention to your scrotum and scan your body for any tension. If you feel tension, get up and move your body or go for a walk until it is gone, then return to the exercise.

3. As you inhale, contract your pelvic muscles to draw your testicles in toward your body. As you inhale, visualize your breath as energy that is flowing toward and filling your testes. Hold your breath for as long as you feel comfortable, and then let it fall out of your body as you release the tension in your pelvic area.

4. Repeat this series for nine breaths. After a break, carry out three to six more sets.

5. Now begin to pull the sexual energy up along your spine, from the base of your spine (root chakra), then to your lower back (sacral chakra). Each time, visualize that center filling up with energy before continuing to move up the spine.

6. Keep moving your energy up your body using this series of breaths, through the navel/solar plexus chakra, followed by the heart chakra, to the throat chakra, the third eye chakra, until you reach the top of your head, your crown chakra.

7. Finally, use one deep, powerful inhale to pull the sexual energy all the way from the testicles to the head. You can do this exercise several times or just once—whatever feels good to you.

The Pink Sparkly Vagina

Most Tantric and Taoist traditions revere the female genitals, or the yoni in Sanskrit (which is directly translated as "sacred gate"), as a major sexual power.

CULTIVATING SEXUAL POWER

One of my favorite ways to demonstrate the healthy use of the yoni's power is with the Pink Sparkly Vagina exercise. This is one of my favorite orgasmic exercises for women. If you have ever struggled to feel love or pride for your genitals, it can affect your ability to reach orgasm and be able to truly enjoy yourself during sex. In a clinical study I performed with KY lubrication, I found that women with poor genital self-image were much more likely to struggle with sexual desire and sexual enjoyment. But when women had a positive view of their genitals, they were much more likely to have a better sex life.

The female clitoris, with more nerve endings per millimeter than anywhere else in the body, is the only organ specifically designed for pleasure. The vulva, or the external part of the female genitals, is filled with blood vessels and nerve endings that engorge and fire with arousal. Your vagina deserves your awe. It deserves your devotion. It deserves your tenderness and gentle attention.

The vagina, your "sacred gate," is powerful. It belongs to a long line of women who have birthed, mourned, loved, lost, and sustained human life throughout all of history. It is the seat of your full divine feminine power.

The key to this exercise is to put all your conscious awareness *inside* your vagina. What does this mean? You will understand if you try it first with something a little less taboo than your lady parts, like your elbow or the tip of your finger. Close your eyes, take some deep breaths and put all your awareness, all your conscious attention, on the tip of your pointer finger. Imagine shrinking your consciousness to a pinprick of light and traveling there. Or if that feels too complicated, just put all your concentration there, even if for a few seconds. This is what I want you to do with your vagina!

SEX MAGIC

1. First, practice alone. Ground yourself and take some deep breaths.
2. Now close your eyes and move all your conscious awareness to the inside of your vaginal canal. Imagine that the walls of the vagina are filled with sparkling, beautiful pink light. Allow the sparkling light to swirl or move in waves. If you want, create a whirlpool of swirling pink sparkling light, filling the vaginal canal. Remember, where attention goes, energy flows.
3. Practice holding this vision and opening and squeezing your Kegel muscles. Notice what that feels like and note your arousal levels.
4. If you are alone, you can stop here, or if you want to take it to the next level, start self-stimulation while you hold the focus of the pink swirling light filling your vagina. As your arousal increases and/or you get closer to orgasm, imagine the light swirling faster and intensifying and spreading out to your labia, even through your body and emanating out, filling the whole room. Your divine feminine yoni energy is infinite and can travel far. Not to mention that sexual arousal and orgasm are some of the highest-frequency energy there is, so spreading out to the world is very helpful! It's not just your partner who enjoys feeling the pink sparkly vagina. You will notice your arousal and orgasmic potential (when alone or with a partner) is much greater when practicing this.
5. If you are having sex with a partner with a penis, get ready to drive him wild during penetration. Imagine your pink, sparkling vagina surrounding and swirling around and bathing your partner's penis. You can even imagine the light squeezing

CULTIVATING SEXUAL POWER

and sucking your partner's penis into your divine feminine vortex. Your arousal will be through the roof too.

Note: It can be fun to practice this without warning or advising your partner about the beautiful, sparkling light you are going to swirl around them. Just do it and watch how they respond. They likely will find the sensations intense and become much more aroused and more quickly orgasmic than usual. And one more thing: If pink doesn't vibe with you, you can picture purple or blue or turquoise. Maybe you want to picture your vagina as a rose, unfolding petal by petal for your partner as they dip into it like a happily buzzing bee. Or maybe you picture your vagina as a warm, salty ocean, filled with all the magic and life of the universe.

And guess what? If you have a penis, you also can harness some energy there! Visualize your penis as an anchor connecting to your partner, as a golden cord of light that helps unite you deeply to the person with whom you are sharing your body. Use whatever visualization works best for you. Just remember to stay with your body and continually come back to putting all your conscious awareness into that region.

The Bottom Breath

This is another great exercise for building internal pelvic sexual energy. Bottom breath moves energy around the genitals and the body in general, and it's very easy to do. It seems simple, but it not only strengthens the pelvic floor for better orgasms, but after ten repetitions, the blood flow has increased to the pelvic region and the baseline for intense arousal kicks in. Do this on its own, or prior to sexual activity to maximize the arousal process.

SEX MAGIC

1. Sit on the floor with your legs crossed or on a chair with feet on the floor.
2. Place your hands on your belly and relax there. Let yourself embrace your body and belly in all its softness and roundness.
3. Exhale the air out of your lungs.
4. Inhale, and as you do, gently push out your anal sphincter. It helps to imagine that your anus is kissing the floor or chair on which you are sitting.
5. As you exhale, simply relax and let go.
6. Repeat ten to fifteen times.
7. It can be a fun exercise to try self-stimulation with your hands or a vibrator while you are doing bottom breath. Notice how the sensations change as you push out your anal sphincter versus when you allow it to relax back into you.

SEX MAGIC CASE FILE

Brandi was the epitome of a Southern belle. She was petite, gregarious, warm, and open. She was the glue that held her family together.

But she began to reveal little cracks in her perfect façade.

As we began working on the challenges in her life, I suggested that she didn't always have to be perfect.

"Tell your husband you're tired of him working late every night. Tell your kids they're old enough to put away their backpacks and lunch boxes. Tell your mom to call your brother at 2 a.m. when she thinks she's having a heart attack for the millionth time that day."

"It's hard to unlearn being the debutante, I guess," she said. "What should I do? I can't do anything you just said. I can't tell my husband

CULTIVATING SEXUAL POWER

what to do, or get on my boys. I can't say no to my mother. I can't even send back a sandwich when the waiter brings me the wrong order."

That gave me an idea.

"Okay," I said. "Let's start with the sandwich."

Starting that day, Brandi and I looked for ways she could start refocusing her yang, or her directive energy. She had the yin down to an art, but she couldn't put a foot down to save her life.

So we practiced in low-stakes situations. She took a deep breath and sent her lunch back when it came with onions. And she told her church friends she didn't have time to do a coffee date that week because she wanted to take a nap instead.

I encouraged her to find ways that she could play with owning her yang energy. How would it feel *not* to reflexively say sorry fifty times a day? How would it feel to put yourself first and not be self-sacrificing?

On Valentine's Day, when she would normally shower her kids with candy and cards and give gifts to their teachers and grandparents, she told the boys they had to make cards for their classmates and teachers. She booked herself a spa appointment and got her nails done. She read a book in the bathtub and ordered a heart-shaped pizza instead of cooking dinner. And something miraculous happened.

"I didn't feel bad for myself. I didn't feel sorry or sad or like my husband or kids didn't love me," she said. "I know they love me. But they don't always show it the way I want. So I am learning to show it to myself, in the hopes that they learn."

And she was right: They did. Her kids made her a Valentine's Day card the next year. Her husband joined her for a couple's massage. They started serving each other instead of her doing all the serving. And all because she was inhabiting her masculine power.

"My husband kind of likes it when I get sassy with him," she says. "He likes me to let him know what I want and what he's doing wrong. I never realized that owning my voice could be sexy and even feminine."

Brandi was stuck in a rut of doing things she hated and feeling like she had no choice. She had to break the cycle. She had to learn how to be a new kind of Southern belle, one who wasn't afraid to stomp her foot and say a bad word every now and then.

CHAPTER 7

Leaving Inhibitions Behind

> Be who you are and say what you feel, because those
> who mind don't matter, and those who matter don't
> mind.
>
> **—Bernard M. Baruch**

nhibition comes from the Latin word *inhibere*, which means to hold in or hold back.

We aren't born with inhibitions. We aren't born holding anything back. As infants, we instantly cried out if we needed milk or warmth or comfort. Nothing about an infant is inhibited. They ardently express their needs without reservation because doing so is key to their survival.

But over time, we learned that our needs might not always be welcome, much less met. We learned that our needs might irritate others. To be safe, we needed to hide our vulnerabilities and keep our softest parts hidden from the harsh light of the world.

While certain inhibitions can help us function in society, many of them, especially sexual and body inhibitions, were born out of trauma ("Big T" or "little t" kind), and a desire to be accepted. But the truth is you are lovable exactly as you are. You deserve to have your needs met. Holding back does not serve you in any way.

Learning to identify and lovingly release our inhibitions is the key to true freedom, especially in our most intimate relationships. I have met couples who have been married for decades who are still shy and inhibited in the bedroom. They've faced every challenge life has thrown at them, they've grieved together, they've grown together, they've built businesses and created children together, but they're still afraid to truly let go in the bedroom. They're still afraid that the person who has been sitting across the breakfast table from them for forty years might judge them if they want to try a new position.

But remember, your inhibitions are not your enemies. They are merely a manifestation of how deeply you desire love—and how deeply you fear you aren't worthy of it.

Follow where your greatest fears lead you and you will be headed toward the growth that your soul is seeking. Toward the reason you are here on this planet, in this dimension, in this body right now.

Once you shift your perception from shame to gratitude, you will discover how much your fear has to teach you. And you will realize that this fear was never fear at all, not at its core. At its core, our fears are invitations. They are sacred opportunities for us to become the heroes of our own stories.

You don't have to slay what you are afraid of. Your fears are not something for you to kill or to overcome. Your fears are your gold, but you need to practice spiritual alchemy to make that transformation possible.

USING YOUR SHADOWS TO FIND THE LIGHT

Your shadows are your greatest gifts. They are the aspects of your personality that cause you the most pain and shame, the places in your

LEAVING INHIBITIONS BEHIND

heart that have been the most traumatized and wounded. But these shadows are your light sources.

As the musician Leonard Cohen so beautifully put it, the cracks are where the lights get in. This is true in your sex life as well. In fact, the more painful and shameful your experiences with sex have been, the more pleasurable and ecstatic your experiences with sex can be.

We often wrongly think that someone with sexual trauma or major inhibitions is never going to be able to wholly enjoy sex. Let me assure you that this does not have to be the case. Many of the people I have worked with who have experienced sexual assault or abuse have gone on to build sex lives that are more deeply fulfilling and joyful than they ever thought possible.

But for this to happen, you can't run from the pain. Our instinct is often to resist discomfort and to flee from anything that challenges us. This is especially true if you grew up in a home where you weren't allowed to display emotions like sadness, fear, or anger. Most of us learned very early on that we needed to be happy and uncomplicated for our parents to be okay.

The truth is that no emotion is bad. Emotions are simply e-motion, energy in motion. They are information. Every emotion can be felt and welcomed on its own terms, including in the bedroom.

Ironically, when we welcome an unpleasant emotion and sit with it rather than fleeing from it or pushing it away, we are more able to fully release it. When we run from it, it sticks to us like glue, never fully leaving us even when we think it's gone.

What is holding you back from being the person you want to be? What fears are keeping you from being the most passionate, most vulnerable, most authentic version of yourself?

I don't believe your fears are an accident. They might feel like an unwanted consequence of childhood trauma, such as the adult who is

SEX MAGIC

afraid of commitment because their parents had a tumultuous relationship. But I promise you that your fears are a gift.

IDENTIFYING AND RELEASING INHIBITIONS

How can you apply this wisdom in your bedroom so that you can have more earth-shattering orgasms?

It starts by attending to your inhibitions.

If you're feeling inhibited in the bedroom, the first thing to do is to figure out what emotion is driving that experience for you.

For example, many women feel inhibited in the bedroom because they don't feel sexy enough or desirable enough. Men sometimes feel inhibited for the same reason, but they can also feel inhibited about whether they can perform well enough to please their partner, or whether they can be vulnerable and drop the machismo act during lovemaking.

Some sexual abuse victims find that they have built a wall of anger, and that anger is telling them to stay hidden or refuse to fully give themselves to anyone ever again. This can also happen with victims of cheating.

So let's explore: What lies beneath your sexual inhibition? Do not be afraid to excavate deeply, because this is where your sexual gifts will be hidden, and the light will enter you.

Make a Release List

Create three columns on a piece of paper. Title the first column "My Stories."

In this column try to list every possible limiting or negative story or belief you have about sexuality and sexual behavior and how they relate to you and your experiences overall. For example, maybe you feel dirty when you masturbate, or maybe you feel ashamed when you identify as heterosexual yet fantasize about the same sex. Or maybe you believe that only desperate women chase after sex, or that men should never say no to sex. Maybe you think you're too fat or your breasts look funny, or you are bad at oral sex.

Then title the next column "From." In this column, write down where those stories originated. Did they come from a specific incident or person? Is it an overall lesson that you were taught at your church or in your culture, such as "Sunday School lessons about puberty" or "Music videos/TV shows"?

It could be something specific, like maybe you are self-consciousness about how your body developed before everyone else during puberty and how that made you a target for bullying. Or perhaps a parent walked in on you while you were masturbating and shamed you about it, or maybe they always urged you to cover up and not dress a certain way because it was dirty or wrong.

Finally, title the third column "K or R." "K" means "Keep," and these are for the stories that you want to retain as you move forward. These are the stories that you feel most intimately linked to, the ones that feel like core values for you. "R" stands for "Release," meaning you no longer wish to subscribe to this story or belief.

I find that when my clients make a release list, it not only helps them identify all the conscious and even unconscious inhibitory stories they've been carrying about their own sexuality, but it also allows them to externalize the messages.

So, for instance, the next time they notice guilt coming up as they perform oral sex on their partner, they can automatically remind themselves, "That's not *me* feeling this way; this is an old belief that I am now able to release," or "There's nothing wrong with telling him

SEX MAGIC

what I want. That's just the conversation I overheard between my mom and aunt when they were calling their other sister a slut for asking her man to go down on her."

Dive into Reality Testing

Beyond coming up with your release list, you likely have some inhibitions or fears around your body and sex that you've developed over time that want to be released so you can fully and freely explore sex magic. Many times, all that's needed is a little reality testing.

For instance, here are some of the common insecurities I hear from people when it comes to sex:

* I won't perform well enough.
* My penis isn't big or hard enough.
* My vagina is too big or loose or smells or looks funny.
* My belly is a turn-off, or my cellulite is gross.

This is where reality testing comes in: a therapeutic, cognitive process through which we can evaluate the accuracy and validity of our thoughts, beliefs, perceptions, and interpretations of the world around us. It's a matter of testing assumptions and determining their validity beyond your own fears.

One of my favorite authors and teachers, Byron Katie, offers a wonderful system for reality testing those negative stories, called "The Four Questions." I have created a variation of my own based on hers. I highly recommend her book *Loving What Is* if you want to explore this further.

Begin by grounding yourself as you learned in chapter 2 to get into your body. Get really clear on the inhibition you want to test.

Then, once you are clear on the story, ask the four questions:

LEAVING INHIBITIONS BEHIND

1. *What is the story I am telling myself?* It can help to write it down so you can externalize it in front of you. Write it as a statement, such as: I am not sexually desirable at my current weight.

2. *Can I be absolutely sure that my story is true?* Hint: The answer (if you are honest with yourself) is no. Can you be absolutely sure that any thought is true? Every single thought is arguable.

3. *What would be the opposite, or a better-feeling story?* Following the example above, this could look something like: I may not be happy with my current weight, but it's just a story I have that this makes me undesirable. My partner keeps saying I'm hot, so I choose to believe him. Regardless of my weight, I commit to remembering that I'm a sexual person who is capable of (and deserves) giving and receiving love and sexual pleasure.

4. *Who would I be and what would I feel right now if the opposite story were the truth?* Really feel into that different story and feel how that story changes your perception, both physically and emotionally.

For instance, a person who wasn't happy with their current weight could imagine what it would feel like to feel perfect just the way they are. While imagining and visualizing how it might feel to love their body, they might respond to their body differently. They might feed, move, and dress their body differently. When our stories change, everything changes, and all that is needed to initiate that chain of events is a willingness to challenge our "truths" and to be curious about other possibilities.

When you apply these questions to your inhibitions, you will likely be surprised to find that the things you think are true are actually false, or at least totally arguable.

Start with Low-Stakes Challenges

It can be daunting to explore sexual activities and behaviors that are out of your comfort zone or make you feel vulnerable. I am a big fan of systematic desensitization, where we progressively and slowly expose ourselves to something scary or uncomfortable. The basic idea is to start with things that feel a little less scary and work your way up. For instance, if you are afraid of anal play but it's something you really want to try, you can get a wax so you are smooth and hairless down there. It doesn't mean you have to leap right into anal, but it can make you feel empowered to know that you are starting to seriously play with the idea.

If you have a rape fantasy but that feels too extreme, try masturbating with your legs lightly entwined as if they're bound. Or blindfold yourself with a scarf. These are ways you can begin to play with how it would feel not to have control. Then you can implement some of those ideas during sex. Ask your partner to hold your arms down during sex or try light bondage.

You can also do these low-stakes activities outside the bedroom too. For instance, if you always wanted to ask a guy out, but typically chicken out because you think women shouldn't initiate, then you can challenge yourself to simply start a conversation with the cute guy on the bus or the handsome neighbor who lives in your building. You don't have to ask them out. You don't even have to flirt. But you can smile and be friendly, and slowly start to dip your toes into the idea that women can lead these connections.

Play with Your Inner Child

We all have a wounded inner child. We never lose this child, or this connection to our past. But our inner child is more than just

LEAVING INHIBITIONS BEHIND

a connection to our past; they are also the gateway to building the future we want to see.

Your inner child might be very quiet. They might not make any noise at all. Or so you believe. But I think you will find that when you start making even the smallest amount of space for your inner child to communicate, you will begin to realize how much you have been influenced by this seemingly silent spirit throughout your life.

As you start to listen to your inner child, you find that the messages come pouring through. It could be very overwhelming at first. Picture a mailbox that hasn't been opened in weeks. The letters and packages will come tumbling down in a cascade when you open it. I find this often happens with people who have done some therapeutic work before. If you've gone to therapy, read many self-help books, or simply been open to spirituality practices and nontraditional healing efforts in the past, you may find that it isn't hard to get your inner child to start talking to you. Sometimes you might even wish that they would be quiet once in a while!

For other people, communication from your inner child could feel slow and hesitant. Your inner child might not trust you or feel safe expressing themselves. I promise you, however, they are listening and waiting. Like a cat hiding under the couch and watching the movement of a visitor, your inner child is determining whether it's safe to come out.

How can you start welcoming your inner child, especially as it pertains to your sex life? Visualizing yourself as a child is a good place to start. Do you have a photo from your childhood that you can pull out of an album or even just scan or take a screenshot of it and print it out? It should be a photo of just you, if possible. You don't have to remember where or when the photo was taken, though it can be helpful if you have positive memories associated with the location in the photograph. If you experienced sexual trauma as a child or adolescent, it would be ideal to try to find a photograph from around that dark time in your life.

Now it's time to start exploring further. Find a quiet time to reflect and connect with your inner child in your mind and heart. Ask questions like those below, and journal the answers, or just hear the answers in your mind. Even better, speak out loud and let yourself have a back-and-forth discussion about their experience so long ago.

Here are some questions to ask your inner child:

* How do you feel about yourself?
* How did you express love?
* How was love expressed to you?
* *Was* love expressed at all?
* Was it expressed in a way that felt safe, or a way that felt intrusive?
* Did you know about sex or romance? Who taught you those things?
* How did the adults in your life express love or sexual desire to each other?
* How did the adults in your life manage romantic disappointment?
* What emotions were you allowed to have?
* What thoughts were you not allowed to express?
* What reaction did you get from your most trusted adults when you shared emotions like anger or sadness?
* How did you feel about your body, especially your most intimate parts?

LEAVING INHIBITIONS BEHIND

* Did you know about consent? What happened when you didn't consent? Did anyone listen?
* Did you get blamed or supported when you spoke out about someone making you uncomfortable?
* Were you believed when you shared your experiences?

These questions are just a starting point. Your inner child will have answers for your questions you wouldn't even know to ask. Hold space for them and let them speak.

What you will find is that your sex life as an adult might be surprisingly linked to childhood experiences that you never even considered. Even beyond trauma and abuse, your sexual pleasure can be impacted by things like your parents' relationship, your culture's approach to sex, the media you were exposed to as a child, and even your first crushes and dating experiences.

Your first sexual experiences can greatly color the rest of your sex life. Research has shown that this is particularly true for women. Women who say that their first sexual experiences were unpleasurable or even unwanted will be more likely to have sexual concerns later in life than women who reported positive and desired first times. Of course, it could partially be that women who had enjoyable experiences early in their sexual life may have had a stronger and healthier upbringing overall, leading them to have better outcomes in adulthood as well.

Regardless of why this is, the fact remains: Your first time mattered. Your initiation into sexual activity mattered. So if your first time wasn't pleasurable or was perhaps even traumatic, that is going to be a part of your sexual experience even now—until you can heal and incorporate those broken pieces of you into your sex life.

BUILDING SEXUAL AUTHENTICITY

Sexual authenticity lives at the intersection of surrender and control. It is where we are our most vulnerable, brave selves, but we are also strongly grounded in our power and our autonomy. We own our sexual pleasure, but we also protect it. We relish the pleasures of the flesh while also inviting our souls to guide and inform these carnal joys.

Sadly, finding examples of sexual authenticity can be shockingly rare. The way sex is portrayed in mainstream movies and in pornography is often completely unrealistic and unachievable. But the good news is that this kind of sex isn't the sex magic that you want to achieve. It is a sham, a sad substitute, and not something worth striving for or emulating.

That doesn't mean that you can't enjoy watching pornography or that pornography can't have a role in a healthy sex life. But just be aware that watching porn can literally rewire our desires and have a negative impact on our sexual response.

That's because even if you think to yourself, "Porn isn't real," or "This is just a movie, it's not real life," it doesn't matter in terms of the neural connections being made in your brain.

Watching porn repeatedly begins to rewire our brains, affecting the way we become aroused and the things that arouse us. Some research has even come out recently showing that when we watch porn, our brains process the objects of our arousal as 2D, not 3D. So we not only become dependent on that visual stimulus for arousal because our brain is looking for the quickest, most efficient way to accomplish the task at hand, but we become programmed to respond sexually to two-dimensional objects, rather than to a three-dimensional person!

Because of the dopamine pathways that are stimulated through watching porn, it's easy to become desensitized and even addicted to it. We get to the point where we need to seek out more extreme (or even violent) pornography to satisfy our arousal desires. None of this is aligned with sexual authenticity, because we aren't even present and fully in our bodies when we are viewing something on a screen. You can't create sex magic when one hand is scrolling Pornhub, or when you are mentally cataloguing the videos you recently watched on OnlyFans. Sex magic is sex that occurs when we fully inhabit every inch of ourselves.

So, while porn can be used as a jumping-off point at times, it can also very quickly become a crutch and even a barrier to intimacy. I advise you to enjoy it, but not too often, and that you do so with your partner (if you have one) rather than alone.

SEX MAGIC CASE FILE

When I first met James over Zoom, he was calling me from his new house in Nashville that he had just bought with his husband, Tom. The newlyweds were in their mid-twenties and pursuing career goals while happily choosing to be childfree. Their lifestyle was high-energy and Instagram-worthy. They took cross-country motorcycle trips, they accomplished triathlons together, they went to electronic dance music (EDM) festivals all over the world, and they enjoyed all the luxuries that come with high-paying jobs and no child-rearing costs.

There was just one problem:

"Our sex life sucks," said James.

We spent time examining James's hormones and lifestyle, but overall there were not any physical or medical reasons why his sex life should be suffering. And he didn't appear to have any depression or mental health concerns that could be a factor either. Other than his sex life, he was feeling very content and happy with his life and with his partner.

What was really going on that was making James feel so disconnected and disassociated in the bedroom?

We began with his childhood, looking at his first thoughts and beliefs about his identity and his sexuality. James said he didn't recall feeling overt shame or discomfort about being gay. He grew up in a liberal family in Portland, Oregon, where he was just one of many LGTBQ+ kids. Even the priest at his childhood parish was openly transgender.

But when we started talking about his first sexual experiences, I began to see a theme. He was almost always watching porn, and lots of it. He reported having sex with porn on in the background, and that he masturbated with online porn several times a day as a teenager.

"My parents are pretty progressive," said James. "It was okay to watch porn. I didn't have to hide it. I could have boyfriends stay over and they were cool with it. I always felt lucky that I never had to feel ashamed to be gay. I knew some people in the world judged us, but Portland was like an oasis where none of that mattered. My parents loved me and always made me feel like I was allowed to be me, whoever that might be."

Whoever that might be. This phrase stuck out to me.

"Did you feel the same way?" I asked him.

"What do you mean? That it was okay to be gay?"

"No," I said. "That you were free to find out who you might be."

He frowned a little. "I think so—wait, what do you mean?"

"It's hard to be 100 percent yourself and present when you're behind a screen," I said. "Your sexuality was established from a voyeuristic perspective. Even when you were having your first sexual experiences, you say porn was playing in the background."

He shrugged it off.

"I'm not addicted to porn," he said. "I barely even masturbate these days."

"No, I don't think you're compulsively using porn. But I do think that you never truly found your sexual self. In fact, I think you're still sort of a virgin."

Here James cracked up for several minutes. I smiled patiently.

"Okay, okay," I said finally. "But I really feel like you've actually never invited yourself into the bedroom. Your body was there but your spirit wasn't. Picture yourself taking a walk in nature. I know you love hiking."

He nodded.

"Okay. Now what if the whole time you were hiking you were looking at your phone and watching videos of other people hiking?"

He scoffed, and then froze for a moment.

"I think you've not only been desensitized to the beauty and magic of sex, but you've never actually fully inhabited yourself. That's why even when you try taboo things like making out with a stranger when you're at a festival you still don't *feel* anything. You're like a powerless, passive observer who's watching your life play out, instead of an active participant who is feeling, experiencing, and creating sensations."

James started to cry. We sat there together for a while.

For the rest of the session, I held space for James to grieve, letting him feel the sorrow of realizing that he had been neglecting this vital part of himself.

Over our next several sessions, we unpacked the idea that all of the high-intensity, adrenaline-pumping activities that he engaged in as a way to *feel* were actually a way *not* to feel, a way to escape the work of being vulnerable and present, a way to substitute drama for connection.

True sexual power has to come from the inside out. Even if you are free of sexual shame and enjoy sexual exploration, you still have to consciously create a space for vulnerability and stillness in the bedroom. Sexual power is not about the risks you are willing to take on the outside, but about the risks you are willing to take on the inside.

CHAPTER 8

Spells and Rituals for Creating Sex Magic

Anything I cannot transform into something marvelous, I let go. Reality doesn't impress me. I only believe in intoxication, in ecstasy, and when ordinary life shackles me, I escape, one way or another. No more walls.

—Anais Nin

Whenever I ask people to tell me about the most amazing sex they've ever had, chances are the word "magic(al)" is included. Not all sexual experiences are magical, but magic can definitely be a sexual experience. Sex, and sexual energy (if you use it right), can be among the most powerful tools of manifestation you possess.

It is said in Tantric traditions that the planet Earth was created when the god Shiva, the god considered to be the embodiment of consciousness, had sex with the goddess Shakti, the goddess considered to be the embodiment of energy. This is the basis of sex magic. You are creating something brand-new out of your sexual energy, alone or when joined with your partner.

The writings about the power of sex to create magic go back thousands of years to the Kabbalah—sacred Jewish texts and teachings—and are found in the Shamanic traditions from around the world.

Using spells and rituals in sexual encounters was first introduced to the Western world by a man named Paschal Beverly Randolph. Born in 1825 a free Black man, Randolph was raised in New York and was a spiritualist, doctor, writer, and advocate for women and people of color. He authored the book *Magia Sexualis*, which wasn't published until fifty years after his death. Randolph called what is now understood as sex magic "Affectional Alchemy." Randolph believed that by working with sexual energy, we could unlock magical powers.

Aleister Crowley is another example of a teacher and alchemist who was attuned to the magical power of sexuality. He lived and taught in the early 1900s and believed that sexuality is at the core of existence and has the power to change the world. He wrote many books on the topic, including one entitled the *Holy Book of Thelema*, which promotes breaking societal taboos around sexuality.

The British occultist Dion Fortune also wrote sex spells, and these were often rooted in her study of the Kabbalah. She saw sexual energy as life-force energy and, in 1924, she wrote *The Esoteric Philosophy of Love and Marriage*. Here she talks about how the sexual energy between two people created during lovemaking can be collected and compressed into a powerful vortex.

The use and techniques of sex spells to manifest our desires lay dormant except among an esoteric, spiritual few. In recent years, more has come out about the technology of using sex for manifestation. Most practitioners believe—and I agree—that it has remained hidden for so long in large part thanks to organized religion. The churches and temples did not want their members to know they could create miracles on their own without their religious institution's support, prayers, or tithings. The religious powers especially didn't want any magic to be discussed or experienced with sex, and it has been touted as "sinful" in almost every context.

Most who practice sex magic spells and rituals do so to supercharge something they want to manifest or bring into reality. But many practice sexual spells and rituals to connect more with their energetic body, connect with the divine, find more erotic confidence, raise their sexual energy as a form of prayer, send up a devotion to themselves, or even initiate themselves in a specific spiritual path they are taking.

USING SEX AS A MANIFESTING TOOL

As we covered in chapter 1, quantum physics has demonstrated that our body's energetic frequency, when matched with intention, creates our reality.

As you can see in the Quantum Lovemap shown in chapter 1, feelings of arousal, joy, and bliss are all high-frequency states in your body. The energy of orgasm is considered the highest frequency the body can hold. The higher our energetic frequency, the more we become a magnet to that which we wish to create. This is how you can use sex to create serious magical manifestations in your life.

Many who practice sexual spells and rituals call this new creation or manifestation the "Magickal Childe." This is obviously not a literal child, although it could be if you wanted to get pregnant. The Magickal Childe is a system of energy created by you—either alone or by joining the energies of you and your partner together. I like to think of the Magickal Childe as a seedling you have planted where something new comes into manifestation.

BECOMING A SEX MAGIC MAGICIAN

If you are ready to start practicing, it's time to let your inner magician shine. It's time to learn how to use the quantum power of your sexual energy to manifest your deepest desires in love and in life.

Here's a checklist to guide you in becoming a great sex magician:

* **Be willing to suspend logic.** Challenge our own perception of reality. A good magician can challenge everything they think they know about sex and everything that they think is true about their partner. They can challenge even their own perceptions of themselves. Every feeling is simply that: a feeling, not a fact. The truth is deeper. And a sex magician is willing to go deep.

* **Be present and observant.** Before beginning any experiment or forming any hypothesis, a scientist will simply observe. This means you must be present and hyper-engaged with what is happening in your body. You're receiving the knowledge your nerves and your senses are sending, and you're learning from those cues. You're taking in the information, without judgment or criticism.

* **Stay grounded and open hearted.** This means that you are embodied and feel safe being vulnerable. You are centered and aligned with your values and yourself. You are open to that which you can't see and willing to stay open in the face of what you can't "prove" or explain.

* **Trust yourself and your partner.** This is a crucial ingredient for a sex magician. You can't experience huge, fluid freedom without knowing that there is a harness of safety holding you and embracing you in perfect protection. A willingness to

relax into one another and your own power is key to creating a pleasure-filled and magic-making sexual experience.

* **Stay flexible but disciplined.** The sex magician also must stay rooted in the awareness that everything is a phase, everything is changeable, and everything can be altered at any moment. Your body and relationship are living ecosystems, and you are their ever-constant gardener. Your garden will go through phases of lush greenery as well as phases of decay. From these dead blossoms, your garden can grow more riotously than ever before. So a spirit of commitment, a willingness to be disciplined, and a wholesome desire for improvement are the most necessary aspects of being a sex magician.

When you are stepping into sexual manifestation, certain steps are crucial to follow for it to work. Sex magic is a result of consciousness (your intention) + energy (your body's frequency). First, it's about getting clear on your intention, or what you want to manifest (also known as your Telos). Then that intention is aligned with sensual and sexual action that moves your body into a high energetic frequency, unlocking the magnetizing power of manifestation magic. In sex magic, the sexual act becomes a "magic wand," channeling the potent, high-frequency energy of sexual arousal to amplify and empower the intention we hold, bringing it to reality.

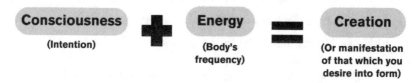

The Equation of Sexual Manifestation

CREATING AN ALTAR FOR SEX MAGIC

One of the most powerful and beautiful things you can do for your sex magic practice is to create an altar. This will be a place in your home that will have the same ability to help *alter* your mood and align your energy with your most heartfelt desires. This isn't like an altar you would find in a church or temple, but one like my client Mercedes created (see chapter 3). You can create an altar even if you are not religious. And your altar doesn't have to be a Wiccan masterpiece or even resemble an altar at all, at least not in the Hollywood sense. It can simply be a meditation pillow on the floor beside a few of your favorite things, things that instantly elevate you to the highest realm of love and joy. Your altar might be outdoors by a bench in your garden. There are no rules here; it's just about creating a space that is *for* you and your highest self.

When you come to it, you are meant to leave differently than when you arrived. The altar is imbued with power because it is charged with the spiritual energy and intention of its worshippers. It becomes sacred and powerful by the intentional acts of worshippers who come prayerfully before it and channel their inner light in this one place, toward this one object.

How to Create Your Altar

There are several items that I have personally found to be beneficial. If you light up at the item mentioned, it's a good indicator that you should have something similar at your altar!

* **Seclusion:** My altar is in a secluded corner in my home office. But I have also been known to take my altar on the go and have sessions outdoors in my backyard or in the forest. You

SPELLS AND RITUALS FOR CREATING SEX MAGIC

need your altar to be your sanctuary, a place where you can be free from the demands of your career, kids, and housework.

* **Crystals:** I have experienced the healing powers of crystals. I believe Mother Earth radiates at such a high frequency that simply being around her majestic rocks and minerals immediately helps me to get into the highest possible frequency. Some of my crystals are gifts from friends or family, which makes them even more precious and full of love.

* **Found objects:** I don't believe in coincidences. I believe the universe is always working to send us little messages and signs. Notice when you come across things like bird feathers, lost pennies, or beautiful stones or shells that speak to you. Save these items and place them on your altar when you come home.

* **Candles:** There is something so soothing and powerful about candlelight. I have several candles that I use during my magical practices. Some people say you should at the bare minimum have a red candle and a white candle for protection, but I say you should just follow your gut and put the candles in your space that feel most necessary to you.

* **Meditation pillow:** You need to be comfy during your manifestation work, and if you're doing manifestation work around sexuality or sensuality, I find it especially helpful to use a fabric that feels yummy and special to you. Choose colors and textures that light you up inside.

* **Tarot or oracle cards:** I love oracle cards. Many people wrongly assume that they are all about predicting the future, but many tarot/oracle card decks aren't geared toward predictions but rather toward helping you discover what your higher self most wants and needs from you. A book of your favorite poetry or religious scripture can elevate you too.

* **Journal or grimoire:** A grimoire is a book of incantations or spells, but I have a grimoire that is simply filled with my experiences of manifestations and rituals. Not every sex magic exercise is going to land for you, but some will, so it is important to keep those exercises on hand so you can return to them whenever you need them. You can also just keep a journal where you write down things you are grateful for or where you collect vision board images or words.

* **Art:** I love the female form and I have many beautiful statues on my altar that feature women's bodies in all their glory. I also have artwork I've made, as well as pieces from friends and family, such as from my father, who was a very talented artist. Again, simply choose artwork that feels inspiring and empowering to you.

CLARIFYING YOUR TELOS

Now that your inner magician is shining and your altar is ready, it's time to get clear on what kind of magic you want to make happen! This is where your Telos comes in. The word *Telos* in Greek means "end purpose" or "goal." In manifestation magic circles, the Telos is an objective you have that you want to bring into manifestation. Are you falling in love? Want your partner to show up in a different way?

Maybe you are hoping to get a promotion at work, or longing for a fulfilling love relationship. The bottom line is that you can manifest just about anything with sexual energy. You can certainly create your own Telos if you are practicing alone or not ready to discuss with your partner yet.

Or, if you have a partner who is participating, discuss your Telos in advance and make sure you agree on what you intend to generate.

The more people generating sexual energy in support of a manifestation goal, the more that goal is supercharged and the stronger the magic is!

When it comes to creating your Telos, it should be as simple as possible, and written as if it's already happened. Your Telos should also be something you can easily hold in your mind. After all, when you are in the throes of passion and arousal, it can be hard to hold on to any complex thoughts!

Here are examples of Teloses some of my clients have made:

* I am orgasmic.
* I win a Grammy for my song.
* I am reunited with my family.
* I write a best-selling book.
* I am standing at the base of Machu Picchu.
* I have given birth to a beautiful, healthy baby.
* I have called in a beautiful love.
* I have a community of like-minded friends
* I am romantically connected to my partner.

SUPERCHARGING YOUR SIGIL

A sigil is a symbol that's created with the intention of manifesting your Telos, your deepest desire. Sigils are encoded with a specific purpose. I like to think of sigils as little seeds we plant. What gives them the power to grow is the energy and intention we put behind them. That's where the magic comes in.

One of the keys to success is being able to simplify your desired goal into a symbol. This is essentially what a sigil is: a symbol of the magic you want to create. It's a kind of shorthand that should capture the full essence of what you are bringing into the world with your powerful sexual energy.

In some ways, images are easier to hold when in deep arousal and left-brained thinking is not operating at full throttle. This is because our subconscious understands the language of symbols and metaphor much better than language. You can look at and hold the image of that which you want to create and subconsciously grasp and hold its meaning, even when you are so aroused you can't remember your own name!

Create Your Sex Magic Sigil

Create your own sigil by following these steps:

1. Do grounding meditation as you learned in chapter 2, and then create an intentional shield around your body. You can create a protective shield by accessing the diamond chakra as you learned to do in chapter 3, and then envisioning a column of beautiful violet or blue purifying light surrounding your entire body. Ask that this shield be a filter that only allows in what is aligned with love and only allows out what you decide you want to release. It is important before doing any kind of magic to set a protective shield, but you can put up a protective shield like this one whenever you wish.

2. Get clear on your Telos, what you want to manifest. Let your mind be open and unfettered. Huge, fluid freedom exists within you and around you. Nothing is off-limits. Nothing is forbidden to you. You can trust where your intuition guides you. You can listen to what your inner voice is telling you. If you are in this space of openheartedness, your intention should arrive to you effortlessly. It will almost be as if your

SPELLS AND RITUALS FOR CREATING SEX MAGIC

heart's desire pops into your mind without your even needing to think about it. It's important to phrase your intention positively, because that is much easier for the unconscious mind to understand. For example, instead of writing "I will not feel anxious when I talk to my partner about money," phrase your intention positively, such as "I feel calm and empowered as I talk to my partner about money."

3. Once you're clear on your intention, live in your body right now as if your desired outcome were already happening for you. It's important to imagine a scenario of that desire as if it's happening right here, right now in the present moment. This moves your body into the energetic frequency of that which you desire. So, for instance, instead of thinking, "I want to be desired by potential mates," you need to think, "I *am* desired by my perfect partner," or more simply "I am desirable" or "I am magnetic."

4. Feel that manifested desire in your body. How does it feel within you when you are desirable? Do you feel a vibrating light in your pelvis? Do you feel a looseness in your shoulders or warmth in your lower belly? Let yourself be with these physical feelings and let your attention make these sensations grow even larger and more defined.

5. Now, write your intention in ten words or less on a piece of paper, again using the present tense, such as:
   * I am deeply desirable.
   * My career is fulfilling and lucrative.
   * I am about to meet the love of my life.
   * I am pregnant.

Once you have written down your Telos, turn it into a sigil or a symbol. Here are the steps believed to work best:

201

1. Look at the written intention. First, cross out the vowels. Then, if you still have a lot of letters (or if you just want to), cross out any repeating consonants (just one of each consonant). For the intention "I am deeply desirable," you would cross out the As, Es, Is, and the Y. Then you would cross out the repeated D and L. Now you're left with MDPLSRB. The goal is to get your manifested intention into as few letters as possible by reducing any excess letters.

2. Form the remaining letters into a symbol. Don't try to preserve the legibility of the letters. Move them around, flip them upside down, and put them vertically instead of horizontally. Your letters don't need to stay looking like ordinary letters. Have fun with this: Be as creative and artistic as you like. Use different pencils or pens to play with color and stroke.

3. Many people like to draw a circle around their sigil to create a safe container for their magical power and intensify the energy.

4. When you're done, you will feel a sense of completion as you look at your sigil.

5. Now charge your sigil with the energy of your Telos. While you hold your sigil, imagine that desired outcome or scenario as if it's happening right here, right now in first person. Feel the energy of the high frequency emotions you will experience when that longing becomes reality and let it run through your body, into your fingers and into the sigil. Like a zip file, imagine the sigil taking in and storing all of that beautiful energy within the image.

I AM DEEPLY DESIRABLE

I̶ A̶M̶ D̶E̶E̶P̶L̶Y̶ D̶E̶S̶I̶R̶A̶B̶L̶E̶

MDPLSRB

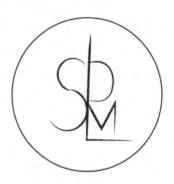

How to turn a manifestation phrase into a sigil

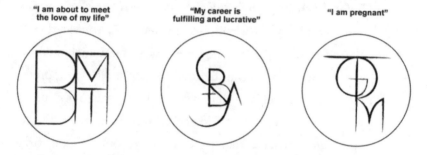

"I am about to meet the love of my life" "My career is fulfilling and lucrative" "I am pregnant"

Some examples of sex magic sigils

Once you feel your sigil is complete, it's time to use it for sex magic! Don't watch porn or listen to music or do anything else that may distract from your sigil. The whole time you're having sex or masturbating, the goal is to remember and continue to think about what you're trying to manifest.

You can watch your sigil with your eyes or hold it in your fingers. Or you can put it on a table or under a pillow. It's just important to keep it nearby so you can have easy access to it during orgasm.

SEX MAGIC

Work with Your Sigil to Create Magic

Manifestation with sex is both an art and a skill. And it requires that you not only learn the techniques shared here, but that you practice them, building up your manifestation muscles.

Once you've made your supercharged sigil, you are going to want to study it and get the image into your mind. Take a picture of your sigil on your smartphone. Keep it handy on your bedside, or wherever you are going to be having sex. There are several ways to use your sigil to create magic during a sexual encounter.

My clients have found these ways the most helpful, but feel free to get creative and think of your own:

1. Before even beginning foreplay, sit quietly on a soft surface and ground as you learned to do in chapter 1. You can do this alone or with a partner. I advise that you are unclothed but you can wear something light and unobtrusive if you prefer. Hold the image of your sigil in your mind or place it in front of you where you can see it. Slowly begin stroking yourself with one finger (or have your partner stroke you), starting from the center of your forehead, down around and behind your right ear, down the right side of your neck, right shoulder, down your right arm and over your right ring finger. Repeat on the left side, holding the image of the sigil as much as you can the entire time. This process has been shown in Somatic Experiencing research to calm the nervous system and access the subconscious mind where we want to imprint the sigil.

2. Infuse the sigil into arousal. Look at and memorize it, then set it aside. As you begin to move into lovemaking or a sexual experience, let the sexual energy begin to build without

SPELLS AND RITUALS FOR CREATING SEX MAGIC

worrying about the sigil, just focusing on what feels good. Then midway into the sexual encounter, when arousal is happening, or even when close to orgasm, pause. If you are doing this with a partner, it will require some communication to let them know when the pause should happen. In a relaxed state just gently gaze at your sigil. After a minute or two, close your eyes and see the sigil in your mind. Now move on and reengage in sexual pleasure, holding that image as best you can while you do.

3. Infuse the sigil into penetration or direct genital stimulation. If you are self-stimulating, imagine the sigil coming onto the tip of your finger or the palm of your hand (or favorite toy) and being placed onto or into your genitals. If you are having intercourse, imagine the sigil attached to the penis (or dildo) and being placed into the receiving partner with penetration. If you are the one doing the penetration, you can imagine the sigil at the entrance of or inside your partner's vagina or anus (or whatever else you happen to be penetrating).

4. Hold the sigil in your hands or hold the image in your mind while you orgasm and imagine your erotic energy flowing into your sigil. Remember, as you learned in chapter 1, where intention goes, energy flows! Picture the energy flowing out of all your pores, or from your heart, or filling you up so much that it expands to fill the field around you. Envision that you are heading straight into the paper and making the letters you created come to life. If you don't reach orgasm, or you can't do this while orgasming, that's okay; just reach for it right after you finish, when your body is still flush with an erotic charge.

Remember, the more intense your sexual arousal and feelings, the more powerful your sex magic becomes. It's really a matter of holding the sigil, or the symbol of your Telos, in your mind, while your body is at an extremely high frequency, sending it out into the quantum field. After orgasm or when the encounter is finished, just relax and enjoy the afterglow while you imagine the sigil in your mind.

Now for the final step in working with your Telos to create sex magic, which is often the hardest. After you have set your intention, clarified your Telos, made a Sigil, charged it with erotic energy, and held the image (literally or figuratively) during arousal or orgasm, it's time to let it go from your mind. It seems counterintuitive, right? It can be difficult to let go and to resist.

GETTING READY TO LET IT ALL GO

This is the final step, and it can feel counterintuitive, right? It can be difficult to let it all go and resist the urge to assert our will upon our circumstances. It requires trust, faith, and patience, all of which can be difficult to come by when we have something we want to see happen. But this is an extremely important step. Remember that it is our high-frequency states while holding the sigil, or representation of what we want to manifest, in our mind and body. After the sexual encounter, your frequency will start to drop some; after all, it is impossible to hold that state of bliss permanently, even if it would be nice to do so.

Furthermore, chances are that if you really want what you are trying to manifest, there is some scarcity energy built in. Just "wanting something to happen" has scarcity built in; maybe it's a feeling of need, or fear (as in "I need this job or I won't be able to pay the bills").

SPELLS AND RITUALS FOR CREATING SEX MAGIC

Most of those things we want badly enough have some fear or even guilt underneath them. For example, if you really want to be sexually desirable and attractive, the low-frequency feeling built in there might be a desire "not to be rejected again." So challenge yourself to find what the hidden dark side of your desire might be.

That's why it's so important to cleanly release the sigil, and the intention, from your mind.

One of the most powerful ways I've found to release one's sigil is to burn or tear it up after you've used it. You can always make another one before your next sex magic session if you want to keep working on the same manifestation. Or perhaps you'll have a new intention the next sex magic session. When you burn or destroy the erotically charged sigil with your desire symbolized upon it, you are releasing it and cannot attach scarcity to it. You can toss your sigil in the fire or in a candle, but please be safe. Dump or bury the ashes—no need to save them because the magic isn't in the paper; it's in you, and in the energy you have manifested. But for now, release it and say, "I am in faith and trust that that which I am calling into me is already in process and I release it and let it go."

BUILDING DESIRE WITH SPELLS

One of the most common complaints I hear from people in relationships is about uneven desire, where one partner wants sex more than the other. I've written about how to treat low and uneven desire in several of my books (*Loving Sex*, *Real Sex for Real Women*, and *The Book of Love*). Most of what I've written about has been focused on the medical, emotional, and relationship strategies for solving the desire issue. But now we can bring sex magic into it! Here is a spell that also helps cultivate desire. All you need is a clear intention and two different colored candles, plus a third white one, along with your favorite scent or oil that makes you feel most sexy. One color candle represents you, the other color your partner, and the white middle candle represents the energy of passion between you.

1. Go to your sexual altar or a comfortable spot that feels safe and sacred. You will need a surface to place the three lit candles.
2. Ground yourself as you now know how to do.
3. When ready, anoint each candle with your preferred scent.
4. In one hand hold the candle that represents you, and in the other hand hold the candle that represents your partner. Close your eyes and imagine the ideal passionate, loving exchange between you and your partner. Imagine it in the first person, as if it's happening right here, right now. You aren't watching yourself in the scene; you are in it. Try to invoke all your senses in your mind's eye. Remember that your body and brain don't know the difference between reality and rehearsal. So when you imagine this way, you are literally putting your body into the frequency of the passionate energy you desire. Do this for a few moments and notice how it feels.
5. Once you have anchored that feeling, imagine pouring it out of your heart chakra and into each candle like a two-way fountain of light. Imagine you are pouring all the feelings you have created in your body of passion and desire into each candle.
6. After a few moments, when you feel you have poured all you can into each candle, it's time to light them. Light the one that represents your lover first, followed by the passion candle, and

ending with the candle that represents you. As the size and intensity of the flame grows, feel heat rising.

If you want your partner to desire you more, say the following:

I have deep, passionate love for _____.
Let _____ desire and long for me as much as I for him/ her/them.
Let his/her/their love enter him/her/them.
Let him/her/them desire me more than they have ever desired before.
Let him/her/them feel the same desire for me that I feel for him/her/them.
Let him/her/them burn with love for me.

If you want to build your own desire, say the following:

I feel deep, passionate love for _____.
Let me long for and desire _____.
Let this love enter me.
Let me desire him/her/them more than I have ever desired before.
Let me feel the same desire for them as much as he/she/they feel(s) for me.
Let me burn with love and desire for him/her/them.

7. Once you are done, allow the energy of the spell to run through you as you sit quietly taking deep breaths.

Make sure to carry out this spell for five consecutive nights to give it maximum power! If you can afford to get five candles of each of the three types (one for you, one for your partner, and one for the energy of passion between you) for a total of fifteen, then go about your business and let the candles burn all the way down by themselves in a safe place. If that's not a possibility, leave the candles burning for an hour or so and then blow them out, saying, "And so it is" as you do.

HARNESSING THE ENERGY OF THE SUN AND MOON TO MANIFEST

Since ancient times, civilizations across the globe have revered the Sun and the Moon as sacred entities, tapping into their mystical energies for spiritual insight and practical guidance. From ancient Egyptian Sun worship to the lunar calendars of the Mayans, humanity has recognized the profound influence of these celestial bodies on earthly affairs. Shamans, priests, and wise women have long conducted rituals and ceremonies to honor the Sun and the Moon, seeking their blessings for fertility, healing, and divination.

Across cultures and epochs, many understand the mystic power of working with the potent energy of the Sun and the Moon. The Sun brings an abundance of solar energy, creating explosive, combustible passion. The Moon tempers this passion with intuitive, connecting energy. Working with both the Sun and the Moon creates powerful passion and connection, especially when matched with a sexual (or even general) intention. This exercise brings the power of the Sun and Moon into your sex life. The only material you need is a candle to light.

1. Stand before the sexual altar you made, or anywhere you feel connected to nature and/or the planets.
2. If you wish, you can intone a sacred word from the Tree of Life in the Kabbalistic tradition that is intended to unite what

SPELLS AND RITUALS FOR CREATING SEX MAGIC

is above (energy, frequency and the spirit realm) with what is "below" (meaning in our 3D reality). This word is *Samekh*. Close your eyes and feel the vibration of the word as you say it out loud.

3. To invoke the passion and energy of the Sun, imagine a yellow-gold spherical ball hovering over your head. Breathe the energy of the Sun through your crown chakra at the top of your head and feel it cleansing, illuminating, and activating every cell in your body, from your head to your toes. Allow yourself to bathe in the healing and activating energies for a few moments.

4. To invoke the cooling and connecting power of the Moon, visualize a silver-white spherical ball above your crown, and as you breathe in imagine the calming, mystical, cooling, and connecting light flowing in and filling every cell. Allow yourself to be flooded with the Moon's feminine grace for a few moments.

5. When you feel filled with the light of the Sun and the Moon, it's time to light a candle and actively call in the power of the Sun and the Moon to you. You can say something like this:

   * **For the Sun:** "Oh beautiful, life-giving, energizing, and activating Sun, I call on you now to bring your passion and activation so I can feel your radiance within me and the alchemy of your erotic activation."

     You can also use the divine name of Tiferet, also the Kabbalistic Tree of Life, representing harmony, beauty, and balance, Yod Heh Vav He Eloa Vada'at. You say it out loud, extending the vowels.

   * **For the Moon:** "Oh gorgeous, intuitive, wise, and illuminating Moon, you who hold the mysteries of the Earth and my subconscious, I call on you to cut through the

darkness and illuminate, cool, and calm my psyche, and connect me more deeply to myself and my partner, fueling our psychic expression and erotic activation within me.

You can also use the divine name of Yesod, also the Kabbalistic Tree of Life, representing harmony, beauty, and balance, Shaddai El Chai. You say it out loud, extending the vowels.

6. Once you feel fully imbued by the energy of the Sun and/or Moon (you can work with either, but I love working with both), it's time to state your now super-charged intention. Here's a script to get you started:

* "I declare that by working with the power of the Sun and/or Moon, I have drawn in their energies to activate my erotic alchemy and call forth the intention of _____. May the Sun's and Moon's energy move through me in this erotic alchemy, for the highest good of all and aligned with the highest frequency. And so it is."

Note: If you are doing this exercise with a partner (or even imagining the partner), you can share one Sun and one Moon big and bold above your heads, bring the energy into each of your bodies and then, once you feel the energy fully inhabiting your bodies, let it get even bigger, expanding out and combining together into one passionate or connecting luminous light. Then you can say the intention out loud together as well to give it the power of both your activated erotic alchemy.

SEX MAGIC CASE FILE

Daniel came to me as a client a few years after a painful divorce. He had met his ex-wife Katie when they were at freshman orientation.

For the next twenty years, they were inseparable: They graduated, went to law school together, bought a house, and raised two kids. They had a seemingly enviable and well-earned "happily ever after," until the unthinkable happened.

Katie told him she was in love with someone else . . . and that someone else happened to be one of his good friends. Daniel's world came crashing down on him. His picture-perfect life imploded.

In the following years, Daniel tried to put his life back together. He focused on his kids and his career. He tried online dating and nights out on the town. He joined a gym, a church, and a co-ed softball league. He was putting himself out there as much as he could, but he wasn't any closer to finding love, or even comfort, in the three and a half years since Katie had told him she wanted a divorce.

Daniel was not a quitter. He came from an Iowa farming town with few opportunities, and his parents were too consumed with never-ending bills and farm work, not to mention their six other kids, to coddle him or give him much attention.

But he went from being that small-town boy on a corn farm to graduating summa cum laude from an Ivy League school. He applied that same can-do spirit to everything in his life, even his broken marriage.

He couldn't get over that he couldn't make Katie stay. The same issue kept coming back. He would meet a woman and have a few pleasant dates, but then she would end it before it truly began or, worse, ghost him entirely.

I suggested a solution that I find works time and time again. "It's magic."

He burst out laughing. Yet this pragmatic, left-brained attorney was not as much of a hard sell on the idea of sex magic work as I would have expected. So together Daniel and I planned a sex altar in his bedroom.

He struggled to come up with a Telos or, I should say, he struggled to find a positive Telos. At first, he suggested things like:

My wife came back to me.

My ex-friend John got hit by a truck.

I don't love her anymore.

I am not in pain anymore.

I got my old life back.

Finally, with my gentle guidance and intuitive soul-work, Daniel came up with:

I wish I could love a woman again.

At first, Daniel felt as though this Telos was much too easy.

"The hard part is making them love me, not vice versa," he insisted.

At our next session, Daniel surprised me. I had asked him to come up with a sigil he could use for his spells, and from the look he gave me as he left my office, I assumed he would struggle with this assignment.

But he came back with something amazing: a hand-sketched picture of a large oak tree being consumed by flames.

"It's gorgeous," I said. "What does it mean to you?"

"I want to feel like I can be burned up in love and still stand there in the flames. I know what you mean now. I want to love a woman again. I haven't been letting myself. I haven't even been close to letting myself. I was just going out to dinner and drinks with any woman who would look twice at me, then I would spend the whole night complaining about my ex-wife and embarrassing myself."

I handed his sigil back to him. "You're ready to start making magic," I said.

SPELLS AND RITUALS FOR CREATING SEX MAGIC

For the next few months, Daniel regularly charged his sigil with soulful self-stimulation. He was intentional about these masturbation sessions: no more Pornhub or mindless masturbation whenever he was bored or sad. Instead, he intentionally scheduled times on his calendar so that he could enter his spells with focused goals and a set plan. As you can see, although we were getting into very esoteric ideas, Daniel was still applying his left-brain, methodical side.

A change began to grow in him. He was still in immense pain at times, but I could sense him moving into this beautiful state of flow. He started making decisions from a place of power, a place of perfect sureness and stability, the oak tree that can sustain anything, rather than rage or desperation.

He quit the softball league and instead started taking drawing lessons. He quit his gym and started taking Brazilian jiu-jitsu classes instead.

Daniel was trusting himself again. And he was trusting the universe again. Love was out there for him. Love was all around him. I suspected (though I didn't say) that it wouldn't be long before he met a woman who interested him.

Not many people would expect a man like Daniel to have been so willing to try sex magic spells and practices, but his willingness to try anything and to stay committed helped him achieve the release and masculinity he had been seeking since his divorce. If he can do it, so can you.

CHAPTER 9

Getting Creative with Sex Magic

Love is an adventure and a conquest. It survives and develops, like the universe itself, only by perpetual discovery.

—Pierre Teilhard de Chardin

Even once you master sex magic, you're still going to have times where your sex life feels uninspired. It's normal to have ebbs and flows.

While there are always emotional and relationship factors that can play into things, low libido is also often physical or medical. Hormones play a huge role in desire, arousal, and orgasm, so any medical condition or age (menopause or andropause) can negatively affect many aspects of your sex life. Lack of exercise and other unhealthy lifestyle habits can cause sexual side effects. Poor circulation and excess can all detract from desire, and if you don't feel comfortable or attractive, you will likely find that your negative body image can also cause you to be less amorous.

It's also important to remember that your medications can impact your desire. Even common prescriptions such as hormonal birth control can decrease your libido. Other medications that can impact desire include antidepressants, antihistamines, anti-cancer drugs, and diabetes medications. While medications are necessary, you can always talk to your doctor about your concerns with sexual side effects and discover if there are other options or things you can do to help increase your libido.

In addition, stress can also lead to low desire because you have less energy for romance and connection. This is why it is so important to find "me time" and to ask for help when you need it. Women often try to do it all, but in doing so, they often end up frustrated, exhausted, and overwhelmed. Make sure to also talk to your doctor about the potential sexual side effects of medications and medical conditions, including other birth control options that might have less of an impact on your desire, such as vaginal contraceptive rings or intrauterine contraceptives.

FINDING SEXUAL SOLUTIONS

Spend some time letting yourself learn what's not working in your life. And consciously stay in a place of "Yes." Be open when it comes to examining what might be blocking or lowering your positive vibrations and energy around sex. Something as simple as too much social media or reality television could be contributing, but it could also be something more painful to ponder, such as a close friendship that is starting to feel toxic or a parenting issue that is draining you and causing you fear.

Now, stay in that place of "Yes," because it's time to look for solutions. My clients typically take one of two approaches toward these solutions. One group is brimming with all sorts of possibilities and paths, while the other is hesitant and wary about anything that sounds too good to be true, even if it's just a simple idea such as getting up thirty minutes earlier each day.

The first group is great at brainstorming but can lack follow-through. The second group doesn't even want to let themselves have an idea that might fail, but once they have a solution they like, they're steadfast in sticking to it.

If you're in the first group, come up with three simple ideas that you can put into action right now. Ideally, it should not involve you needing to buy anything or begin any massive projects. It should be easily achievable but require follow-through. Examples include:

* Kissing your partner for ten seconds every day.
* Reading an erotic novel before bed instead of scrolling Instagram.
* Spending fifteen minutes every day on something that makes you feel sexy, whether that is dancing or painting your nails or lifting weights.
* Giving your partner one compliment a day.
* Giving yourself one compliment a day (out loud and to the mirror if possible!).

Remember, don't try to reinvent the wheel. Small changes made on a consistent basis are what will make the most impactful changes to your relationship and your sex life.

If you're in the second group, come up with twenty ideas. No, really. What are twenty things you can do that will spark more passion and joy in your life right now? This is a long list, but I want to work on engaging your creative mind and forcing yourself to stop seeking perfection. It's okay if your ideas are not sustainable. You just need to get some thoughts down on paper and start flexing your "it's okay to have bad ideas" muscle. Once you've done this, you should have at least three ideas on your paper that seem largely doable, even if you're fearful that you might not have perfect follow-through. That's okay. The spirit of the intention is what counts.

This exercise can easily help to spark some real changes in the bedroom. Consistently commit to looking for ways to feel sexy every day (and to make your partner feel sexy every day), and it will soon become second nature

MAKING SEX MAGIC IN A KINKY WORLD

By now you have learned how to have soulful, authentic, vulnerable, and present sex. But what if you also want to have dirty, kinky sex that features all your favorite toys and fantasies?

Sex magic can absolutely be kinky. Check out the following ideas for some edgier sex acts and try one, try a few, or try them all! Take your time and remember to communicate, communicate, communicate. When we play at the edge, we need to make sure that we are getting constant feedback and consent. Playing at the edge might feel scary at times, but it should never be terrifying or go too far for comfort.

Most important, when playing with kink, you must be clear on a safe word. When we are exploring our erotic edges, especially with things that may be painful or humiliating, it's easy to accidentally go too far. Safe words should be something you wouldn't normally say in that scenario, like "banana" or "laundry." A safe word lets your partner know that you have had enough and it's time to stop. You may choose to keep going after that, but you certainly don't have to do so. The

GETTING CREATIVE WITH SEX MAGIC

most important part is that consent is constantly being given and both of you feel safe!

Semi-Public Sex

Have you ever fantasized about being watched while you make love? Exhibitionism, or being "caught in the act," is a common fantasy that you can explore with your partner safely. You don't want to run afoul of the law or truly put yourself in danger, but you can play with the idea of possibly being discovered. Public sex would include having sex in front of people or doing it in a public bathroom or park (although you'd get in trouble for public indecency). But you can also explore semi-public sex by keeping the blinds open in your bedroom or enjoying foreplay or heavy petting in your backyard. Have sex in your car (in a safe location) or make out in the movie theater.

There are lots of ways to explore this kink that won't put your intimacy on display. Ask yourself what about this act feels so thrilling to you. Is it that it feels taboo? Is it that it feels sexy to be so desired that your partner can't wait until you are in the privacy of your bedroom? Find out what makes this kink so sexy to you and find ways to awaken that feeling without exposing yourself. Remember, consent is key, including from your partner and the public—you don't want to impose your kink on people who haven't consented.

The Art of Edging

Edging is the practice of delaying orgasm, with men in particular (or those with a penis). Instead of releasing sexual energy right away (or practicing retrograde ejaculation, as you learned in chapter 2), you keep building and building its intensity. This allows not only for more powerful orgasms when you finally do reach a release, but it also allows you to be more intentional and present about your sexual response. It's also important to note that edging is a fantastic way to gain more ejaculatory control for men who want to last longer! Remember, if you have a female sexual partner, women take on average about twenty minutes to reach orgasm while men only take seven and a half minutes! Edging is a wonderful way to close that orgasm gap.

Edging is about consciously working in that sweet spot between excitement and that point of no return. The best way to master edging is alone first, during masturbation. This is a good way to quiet your mind and be able to pay very close attention to your sexual response without distractions. Once you get a grasp on the practice of edging, you can then start enjoying it with your partner.

1. Ground yourself in your body. Do an internal body scan and seek out any areas of tension or discomfort. Keep your body scan going as you start to pleasure yourself.
2. Now start self-stimulation. Using a scale of 1–10, pay attention to where you can feel very excited and aroused without losing control and sailing straight into orgasm. As soon as it starts to feel good, like a 3 out of 10, take a brief pause. Practice slowing down and building your arousal and gaining control.
    * Take deep slow breaths.
    * Slow down a bit or even stop.
    * See what happens when you touch different parts of your body. Can you stay at a 6 or below if you just rub your nipples or stroke other spots?

GETTING CREATIVE WITH SEX MAGIC

* Squeeze your Kegel muscles.
* For men, when you get to about an 8 or 9, squeeze the base of your penis with one hand.
* When you get to an 8 or 9, push into your perineum (the area between the scrotum or vaginal opening or the anus) with your pointer, middle, and ring fingers. Instead of pressing into your perineum with your fingers, you can also utilize the half lotus yoga pose, where while sitting upright, the heel of one foot is under your buttocks pushing into your perineum.

3. Continue to play with increasing and decreasing arousal. See if you can move between a 5 and a 7, touching an 8 and maybe even a 9, and then moving back to a 5.
4. When you finally surrender and allow yourself to go all the way to a 10, get ready for an extremely powerful and intense release!

Once you have mastered edging on your own, practice edging during sex with your partner. All this practice in ejaculatory control will make you an amazing lover! You can use the same techniques you learned previously. Or when you are climbing to 7 or 8, you ask your partner to slow down or switch up your foreplay. You can even go back to making out or spend some time pleasuring each other to bring your arousal down to a level where you can better control it.

Remember, the goal of edging is not just to delay orgasm as long as possible. It's about learning to enjoy the dance of longing, to get lost in the journey instead of just racing to the next destination. It's about being present and engaged with all your senses and turning orgasm into an act of creation rather than competition.

Role-Playing

There are so many titillating role-playing scenarios you can act out. Consider:

* Doctor/patient: Your doctor will see you now—all of you.
* Professor/student: Someone is going to fail unless they are willing to do a little extra credit!
* Boss/employee: Are you going to pass your performance review? You might need to show your commitment to the company—on your knees!
* Domestic discipline: Spanking and time-outs might be in order for the naughty partner.
* Free use: What if your partner could touch you or make love to you whenever they wanted? Many people enjoy free-use fantasies, in which they are doing household chores, watching TV, using the telephone, or the like, and they suddenly find themselves having their clothes ripped off. A common part of this fantasy is that the person just keeps on doing what they were doing, almost ignoring their partner's randy overtures while they use your body to their heart's content.
* Nonconsensual consent: No, it's not an oxymoron. Nonconsensual consent is when you or your partner pretend to be nonconsenting, even though you really are. (Make sure you have a safe word ahead of time so you can call a time-out if you really do need to withdraw consent.) This might look like a rape fantasy in which your partner breaks into your bedroom, or you might pretend to be asleep or incapacitated while he has his way with you. And remember, men enjoy rape fantasies too. Taking him against his will can make him

feel incredibly desirable. (Please note: No one *ever* actually wants to be raped or touched against their will. This is fantasy, not reality.)

Whips and Paddles

Explore your spanking fetish by incorporating ticklers, paddles, crops, and floggers. (Yes, they are all different!) A tickler lets you tease your partner with feathers while also offering a hint of pain when used to spank. Paddles are self-explanatory, but they can come in a variety of fabrics and sizes. Fabric-covered paddles are a good idea for beginners, while experienced spankers and spankees may want to try an acrylic paddle. Just remember to always keep the paddle *flat* so you don't hurt your partner.

Crops are a good option, especially if you are interested in horse role-play. Crops can be lush and beautiful, and even downright feminine and delicate. You can find crops that have a tiny heart shape or crops that are made with leather and lace.

Floggers are similar to crops but they feature the signature cat-o'-nine-tails for extra pain and pleasure. But don't be intimidated: Floggers don't have to be scary. You can choose lightweight options that have soft, velvety fabric instead of rough straps.

Always start slowly and be sure to vocalize what is going on with you. If you're the spankee, tell your partner how you're feeling and if it is getting too hard—or not hard enough. If you're the spanker, constantly check in and make sure your partner is enjoying themselves. And don't forget aftercare! Use soothing lotion on your partner's bottom when they are done being spanked, and make sure to offer lots of pleasure along the way.

Hot Candle Wax

Nothing perfectly walks the line between pleasure and pain like hot wax. But you don't need to use regular candle wax anymore. There are now candles specifically made for use in the bedroom. Many are made with eco-friendly ingredients like essential oils and skin-softening jojoba. They burn at a low temperature so the wax is "Ohhh" hot, but not "Ow!" hot.

Light the candle and let the wax start to pool and soften as you enjoy foreplay. Then, while pleasuring each other, tip the candle slightly to let the wax drip temptingly all over each other. Romantic and kinky all at once.

Sensory Deprivation

Imagine this. You're blindfolded and you can't move your arms or legs. You can't see a thing, nor can you hear. You are wearing a pair of noise-canceling headphones. You might even be gagged so you can't make a sound. Now all your senses—except your sense of touch—have been taken from you.

All of a sudden you feel hands exploring your body and touching you everywhere. You can't resist or control what is happening to you. All you can do is lie back and enjoy the ride.

Does this sound exciting to you? If so, you and your partner might want to play with sensory deprivation. All you need is a blindfold, headphones, and gentle bondage gear. You can even lightly tie your partner up with a pair of panties or a soft scarf. Then let the exploration begin!

Sex Furniture

From swings to pillows to harnesses to poles to spanking benches, sex furniture is a market that every couple should explore, such as:

* Bungee chairs or bounce squatters: These sex chairs work for couples and solo play. If you fantasize about things like face sitting during oral sex but you're not able to hold the position or you just want to be extra comfortable, chairs like this can work for oral sex, manual sex, and penetration.
* Spreading bars: A favorite of BDSM lovers that keeps the arms away from the body and the receiver relatively powerless.
* Sex slings: If you want to experiment with sex standing up but don't have the muscle strength to last in that position indefinitely, try a sex sling that works over your door. It's easy to set up and take down and will let you try a variety of positions that might not be accessible to you otherwise.
* Wedges and ramps: Sex pillows will let you get even deeper and closer. Pillows like this will let you explore tons of new positions or even just bring a new level of pleasure to standard positions like missionary.
* Sex swings: Many sex swings are now easy to install and are a discreet addition to your bedroom, so you don't have to feel like your bedroom has to be hidden behind lock and key if you have guests.
* Spanking benches: If you enjoy spanking and playing with pain and pleasure, these comfy benches will make you feel like you're starring in your very own *Fifty Shades of Grey*.

Food in the Bedroom

Have you ever seen the *Seinfeld* episode where George Costanza tried to incorporate food into the bedroom? It's a sexy idea, but not when it's a pastrami sandwich!

Instead, think ice cubes, whipped cream, edible panties, flavored condoms, edible body paint, chocolate syrup, or honey dust. Whether you're shopping at a traditional grocery store or a sex toy store, there are so many ways you can indulge your sense of taste in the bedroom.

Just one caveat. Be careful about placing foods made with sugar inside the vagina because that can lead to a urinary tract infection. Try sugar-free products instead.

BUILDING YOUR SEX MAGIC FANTASY WORLD

For couples, I always love encouraging the creation of a "Fantasy Box."

* Each of you takes some time to create a list of all the fantasies you can think of that you'd like to act out together. It could be toys or positions you want to try, role-plays, or other things you'd like to explore. These are fantasies, not reality, so let your imagination run wild!

* Sit down together to go over your lists. This will be a beautiful opportunity to learn so much about each other that you may have never known before. It's crucial to make a very clear agreement first that you will not judge each other for your fantasies, even if they feel scary or weird to you. You don't have to do anything that makes you feel uncomfortable, but if you want true intimacy in a relationship, you must allow each of you to present your truest sexual selves.

GETTING CREATIVE WITH SEX MAGIC

* Negotiate a master list. On this list are all the fantasies you agree you'd both like to explore. This may require negotiation. For instance, one of you may want to have sex in a public park, but the other would never be willing to do so. Instead, perhaps you have sex in the backyard in the dark where the neighbors could (but likely won't) see what you are up to.

* Once you have your list of shared fantasies, set an intention to try one of these fantasies once a month. Don't wait for your partner to initiate: You can take the reins here because you'll have all the information you need about what they most desire in the bedroom. And don't let yourself get caught up in the accessories and the shopping. You don't need to spend lots of money to fulfill a fantasy.

If you are single, experiment with different kinks you enjoy on your own. You might read BDSM erotica or buy a new sex toy, or experiment with masturbating with the shades open or writing a short story featuring a rape fantasy. Let your imagination run wild and consider this your time to liberate yourself from your past beliefs about who you are in the bedroom. You can completely rewrite your sexual persona. Just be careful about exploring kink with new partners because it's best to introduce these acts after you have established trust and intimacy. So while you might enjoy chatting on a BDSM website with other like-minded people or even going to a BDSM club, remember to proceed with extra caution and put your safety first. Fantasy should never put your life or well-being at risk.

SEX MAGIC CASE FILE

Faith was a twenty-five-year-old nurse who came to me seeking help for painful sex.

"It all started a year and a half ago," she said. "It came out of nowhere . . . I've been having sex since I was fourteen years old, and it never felt remotely painful before."

After breaking up with her college boyfriend, Faith was happily single and enjoying her twenties. Except recently, Faith noticed that she was having discomfort and even sharp pain during intercourse.

"It doesn't matter who I'm with or how turned on I am," she said. "Sometimes I have to ask my date to stop, or I try a new position, but it doesn't help. It's getting really frustrating."

After making sure Faith didn't have any underlying health or medical issues that might be causing her pain, we started examining when the pain started.

"What have you done to treat it?" I asked. "I mean, what do you do when the pain starts?"

"I usually just try to grin and bear it," she said. "Sometimes I fake orgasm or go overboard with the moaning and dirty talk to make him hurry up and come too."

As we explored deeper into Faith's history, I discovered she had quite a bit of trauma around sex, including childhood sexual abuse and a horrific incident of revenge porn in which a high school boyfriend shared her nude photos with his friends. However, she was adamant that these experiences didn't mar her enjoyment of sex or men.

"I fucking love sex," she told me. "I am not going to let anyone take that away from me."

She said this almost defiantly, and I heard in her voice a quiet, broken desperation. She had fought so hard to own her sexuality even in the wake of the trauma she experienced.

"I am not a prude or some frigid bitch," she said. "I love sex. You should see my nightstand drawer. I have more toys than you do in this office!"

GETTING CREATIVE WITH SEX MAGIC

I laughed. "Well, that must be a lot of toys!"

"For real, though," she said, "I've done things that make my friends blush. I even have a few videos on OnlyFans. They don't show my face, though. I can't because of my job . . . but maybe someday I'll quit and be a full-time porn star!"

Interested, I asked her when she first posted her videos on OnlyFans.

"About a year and a half ago."

"And when did your pain during sex start?"

"About a year and a half . . . wait, what are you saying?" she said. "My videos don't have anything to do with that. It's just me masturbating and having fun. I haven't done them in a while because of the pain, but I think it's so hot knowing strange men are out there watching me."

"I think that is definitely true for you on some level," I said. "You are very adventurous and seem to enjoy a little exhibitionism. But considering what happened to you in high school, I wonder if that triggered something for you. You were a child having explicit photos of you spread around your school. You had no control over that situation. Now, you're creating a similar situation, except you have the control."

"Exactly," she said proudly. "I told you. I've never let that stuff hurt me or keep me from enjoying sex."

She was confident and at ease with herself. Unlike some of my clients who are shy and almost embarrassed to talk about their anatomy or sexual experiences, Faith seemed to revel in the details, and at times I almost sensed she wanted to shock me.

But I knew there was something bubbling underneath that façade that seemed to be daring men to hurt her and daring the world to try to break her.

"I think your vagina is mad at you," I said.

Faith started laughing.

"I'm serious," I said. "You can act as hard as you want and fool the rest of the world, but you aren't fooling Her."

Faith's smile faded.

"There is a part of you that works really, really hard to keep you okay," I said. "A part of you that wants you to love life, to love sex, to be the brave and confident woman you want to be. She works really hard for you. But there's another part of you too . . . a part that deserves softness. Tenderness."

I knew we needed to ease into this trauma and today was not the day. I asked Faith what kind of music she liked. She seemed surprised but told me her favorite singer. I asked her if we could have a dance break. I put on "Dancing Queen" by ABBA and started modeling for her how to shake and move our bodies to shift. My true intention was not only to shift the energy and help Faith get unstuck, but to begin to somatically help her come back into her body.

Again she cracked up but she was on her feet before I was.

This was the first of several sessions Faith and I had together over the next six months. During our time together, I asked her to refrain from sex altogether, which was difficult for her. Self-stimulation was allowed, but, for the first time since she was a teenager, Faith was celibate.

It took about five sessions for Faith to allow her aching, crying child self to come out of its hiding spot. It happened in a very painful way. It was her grandmother's eightieth birthday celebration. Faith was essentially raised by her grandma, and she was very excited for her party. But then she found out that her mother invited her older step-cousin, the man who molested her when she was seven years old.

Faith was shocked and enraged. She hadn't seen the man for many years, but he was recently out of jail (for a different crime) and back in the family picture.

GETTING CREATIVE WITH SEX MAGIC

Faith was quiet that day, quiet for the first time since I had met her. Her body was still and soft. She looked like a puppy who had been kicked. My heart ached for her.

"What were you like when you were seven?" I asked.

"Loud," she said. "Crazy. My mom said I was fast, you know what I mean. Always flirting."

"Flirting?" I said. "Children don't flirt."

Faith looked at me, confused.

"No, that's what they all told me," she said. "I liked to dance and twerk even then. I was always showing off."

"Faith, the little girl that you were then is still in the room with us right now. She's inside of you right now. And she knows what you're saying about her isn't true. She's hurting."

Faith stared at me.

"What were you like?" I asked, and I pulled out one of the childhood pictures she had brought to a previous session. In the photo, Faith had long braids and a giant, goofy grin on her face. She was holding a popsicle and had her arms wrapped around her younger sister.

Faith looked at the picture and dissolved into tears.

"Move your body," I said. "Listen to it. You know what to do."

She seemed to hear me, and soon she lay on the floor, in a fetal position. She clutched a pillow around her stomach. I sat beside her and gently witnessed this amazing birth.

Finally, she began to speak.

"I loved Barbies," she said. "I loved Janet Jackson. I was the best roller skater on the block."

"What else?" I asked.

"I was confused a lot after . . . after he started touching me. I was disgusted by myself, but I also liked his attention. I knew it was bad to be fast. I knew good girls didn't like that stuff," she said. "I was sad a lot. But I knew not to show it. My grandma needed me to be her good girl. I was the oldest. The strongest."

Faith was silent for a moment.

"When I finally told my mother, she was so angry at me," she said. "She blamed me, I could tell, even if she didn't exactly say it. My grandma didn't want to talk about it at all. It just wasn't something her generation could handle, y'know?"

"But you still told."

"I saw him eyeing my little sister in the same way he eyed me," she said. "I had to protect her. I wish I hadn't, though. Because he ended up getting picked up a few months later for a drug charge. So he would have been out of the picture anyway."

"You did a brave, selfless thing. You sacrificed yourself to make sure your sister was safe," I said.

Faith agreed. "I guess so," she said. "But now look what's happening. They all don't care that he's coming to the party. My sister feels for me, but she still sees me as the fast one. They all do. After what happened when I was fourteen, when I sexted my boyfriend, it just felt like I proved them all right. I had to go to an alternative school after those photos came out. My pastor asked my grandma to stop bringing me to church because it was distracting the boys. It was like everyone just gave up on me then."

This is a common story in families with sexual abuse. The child who is abused is often labeled as being the problem, not only for the initial abuse itself, but for the emotional fallout that comes afterward. Often families want the victim to stop being a victim, to stop being in pain. They want the issue swept under the rug. They want the perfect family façade and holiday parties without the stress of confronting the deep, dark trauma in their past.

GETTING CREATIVE WITH SEX MAGIC

In this way, the victim often becomes the black sheep. Because she is the truth teller. The pain holder. The lone outrider who is calling out the problem and asking people to do the hard work involved with healing.

"How am I supposed to forgive them?" she asked me.

I told her she needed to forgive herself. I reminded her that she had been a good little girl and should never should have been touched like that. I told her she never should have had her trust betrayed by her boyfriend and that her family should have protected her and cherished her.

"You've abandoned that hurt little girl because that's what your adults taught you to do. They didn't show you how to be gentle and compassionate with her. But you can. You can break the cycle."

Thus began Faith's journey toward softness. For the first time in her life, she let herself be vulnerable. She protected her child-self by not going to her grandma's birthday. Instead, she took her out to lunch the week after. They didn't talk about what happened. They talked about her grandma's life and what it was like growing up in the '60s. Faith realized that being a strong woman was a role that the women in her family all handed down to each other. That they lived by survival instinct, afraid to soften or be emotional because it didn't feel safe to do so.

Faith's softening took time. It looked different day to day. She took down her dating profiles and her OnlyFans videos. She started a new nighttime routine of hot tea and a book in bed, instead of surfing Tinder. She started a yoga practice and joined a local women's group for sexual abuse survivors. Over time, she began dating again. But her sex life wasn't the same as before. She didn't feel the need to jump right into bed, or to be the kinkiest, wildest one in the bedroom.

"Don't get me wrong, I am still so kinky," she laughed. "But I say no to stuff now. Like, I don't like anal sex, and I used to just force myself to do it. I'd have some drinks and just go with it. But now I don't. In fact, did you know sober sex is actually amazing?"

I laughed and agreed.

The pain during sex took time to slowly fade. We soon realized that she was carrying a good deal of tension throughout her whole body, including her vagina, and this led to that stabbing pain during intercourse. We did somatic therapy and helped her move that locked trauma out of her body. I sent her to work with a pelvic floor therapist, who helped her train herself to tighten and release her pelvic floor muscles as she desired. She learned to release and relax during masturbation, then applied that technique with her partner when she began dating.

And she started writing poetry. Perhaps the most beautiful moment was when she shared (and gave me permission to share) the poem she wrote for her younger self.

> To the little girl who had to become a warrior,
> Who carried the weight like the "fast" girls before her,
> Who learned to clench her fists instead of crying,
> Who learned to pirouette on broken glass and roller-skate through a house on fire,
> Who asked for nothing and got even less—
> Now I will give you everything. Now I ask for everything.
> All the softness, all the gentle words,
> All the "good girls" you never got.
> Now when you call out, I gather close, I pause and breathe.
> Your words grow louder like a rushing wave,
> And I realize you are singing a song I used to know:
> A song of Faith.

CHAPTER 10

Pleasure for a Lifetime of Sex Magic

> For one human being to love another, that is perhaps the most difficult of all our tasks . . . the work for which all other work is but preparation.
>
> **—Rainer Maria Rilke**

ove (like great sex) is an art. And like all art, it is something that we innately know how to do but also a skill we must learn. We are love and we were born with love, yes, but it is a skill. It is a craft. It is never finite or finished.

Just a few last thoughts to guide you on this journey.

First, remember mastering sex magic doesn't mean that your sex life will always be epic and flawless. Even if you're an experienced marathon runner, you're going to have days when your speed is slower than you would like or your gait feels off. A master chef still has recipes that don't always pan out as hoped.

Bring patience, compassion, and even humor to sex. Your relationship doesn't boil down to just the last time you and your partner had sex. It doesn't even boil down to the last twenty times you had sex. Your relationship is so much more than any one encounter. And to accept these ebbs and flows gracefully is not to give in, but rather to become empowered to fix what we can and release what we can't.

The truth is that most of us will get bored with our sex life at certain points in our lifetime, whether in a relationship or not. And this is especially true if you are seeking the intensity you crave from sex outside yourself. When sex begins to feel lackluster, you begin imagining it's something to do with the way you look, the people you are attracting, or your partner.

When you feel bored and unloved in your relationship, the natural impulse is to blame your partner. Maybe they don't pay enough attention to you, or they aren't exciting enough. They don't have a high enough libido, or they aren't interested in trying new things. Or maybe you simply blame the nature of your choices: you've been together too long, your kids took over your life, or you have too many financial concerns, for example.

But our disconnection and boredom with sex—and often with our partners—is almost always because we've lost touch with our own internal world and are seeking validation, connection, and excitement outside ourselves in another. Of course, we need another person to have coupled sexual experiences and to be in a relationship. But after thirty years working to help individuals and couples learn to love and be loved better, I can promise you the excitement, intimacy, and even change you seek begins within you.

SEX MAGIC AS THE ANTIDOTE TO BOREDOM

To me this is the coolest part of sex magic.

You never have to get bored. Sure, you could become so familiar with the intricacies of your body's energy centers and how to move with and use them that it becomes commonplace. You could learn all these exercises so they become second nature. But sex magic calls us to the deepest parts of ourselves, to discover the universe of our internal energy and the energy of which we are made.

Every time you tap into your own internal energy, you open a door to a new experience. As you learn to move energy through your body, build sensations of arousal, and even move them between you, it's impossible not to be amazed at your experience.

There is an endless source there, a cosmos within us, the terrain of which could take a lifetime to explore.

I've been married for twenty-plus years, but in so many ways I am a completely different woman than the one my husband married. And he is a completely different man. Our experiences, discoveries, and longings shift and change over time. In order for your relationship to survive, especially for it to thrive, we must be willing not only to allow for shifts and change but to welcome them. This leaves more and more to discover within ourselves and each other. It allows us to be fully present and vulnerable with ourselves and each other for who each of us are, the universes inside us, rather than what we expect or "signed up for."

Even when we are newly dating, we see what we want to see. Every moment, we are inundated with information, but we see only a fraction of the truth because we are looking through the lens of our own expectations.

There is so much more space and curiosity available to you when you consider the idea that everything you think and assume about your partner and your relationship might be just a speck in a vast universe of possibility.

You might feel an expanse in your chest or a relaxing of your shoulders. Things feel lighter, don't they? And also more exciting.

IF YOU'RE IN A COMMITTED RELATIONSHIP

Perhaps you just haven't been aware that you're using a flashlight instead of turning all of the lights on. You've been in almost complete darkness when there's a kaleidoscope of colors exploding all around you.

If you want to access that excitement, you just have to bring awareness to the fact that everything is possible. When we say, "Our sex life is boring," or "My partner is so unromantic," or "My partner is never in the mood," you have not only removed the possibility from your relationship, but you have cast your partner and you in iron-clad, uneditable roles.

You're both partners stuck in a dead-end sex life without any passion or pleasure. Feel how your chest tightens and your stomach clenches at that thought. See the way your energy and perception narrow. You've become fixed in a story and you have fixed yourself and your partner into roles that you can't escape.

This is why simple awareness and wholehearted curiosity are the greatest tools in your sex magic toolbox. With them, you can challenge any story and rewrite any that no longer serve you. So instead of being locked into the belief that your sex life is boring, or that monogamy is never going to be as "fun" as when you were single, you can choose new beliefs.

Discover this new story about monogamy: You get to spend the rest of your life learning to have passionate, heart-stirring sex with your partner, and you get to be compassionate and patient during those times when it's not everything you might have hoped for. You get to make love anew every day, and find new ways to express that love, and you can do so in a place without judgment or fear or doubt. You get to love and be loved in the most perfect way that two human beings can love each other, and you get to do so for as long as you both have breath in your lungs.

PLEASURE FOR A LIFETIME OF SEX MAGIC

Monogamy? Boring?

We can move beyond our fixed stories about ourselves, our relationship potential, and our partners when we realize how limited those stories actually are. Neither you nor your partner (nor your dynamics) are set in stone. You are meant to be expanding your perception of each other and your perception of love and sex.

Sex becomes lackluster and disappointing when we start to unconsciously box ourselves in and let ourselves be influenced by stories about who we think our partner is or about who we think we are or about what we think relationships should look like over time.

The best thing you can do for your love life is to start every day with the realization that your partner isn't the same person you slept next to last night. Your partner isn't the same person you married or committed to, and your relationship isn't the same as you envisioned when you first thought about love and marriage as a child. And neither are you.

Everything is always changing and anything is possible. You can roll over and start stroking your partner's genitals first thing in the morning, even if you never initiated sex that way before. You can walk around the house naked even if you usually never let your partner see you without your clothes on. You can make out with your partner in the middle of a movie even if you have been together twenty years and you barely kissed each other for the last eighteen of those years.

At any moment, you have unlimited power. You have the power to perceive what you want, to feel what you want, and to create more of those feelings for yourself.

Isn't that exciting?

Yes, I know what you're thinking: My partner is going to think I have lost my mind if I suddenly start doing all of these out-of-character things. Good. Great. Let them think that, because you have. Because sometimes you have to lose your (old) mind to find your soul. And as you continue living this way, your partner is going to find themselves hopping on that ride even if they don't realize it. They will entrain to your energy. They will sense that the rules have changed. That there are no hard and rigid rules anymore. That they can be whoever they want at any moment and that they can take big risks and be vulnerable and messy and bold right alongside you.

As we delve deeper into the recesses of our being, we begin to understand that love and intimacy are not static; they are dynamic, ever evolving, and endlessly fascinating. They thrive on the curiosity to learn and understand, to peel back the layers of vulnerability and expose the raw, unfiltered truth beneath.

This adventure of love is the accelerant that will keep the flames in your bedroom going. This is the way you never have boring, meaningless sex again. This is how you engage in and have true sex magic.

I firmly believe that our partners are our greatest teachers. Our soulmates are put here not only to love us, but to trigger us. They trigger our deepest wounds and are often a mirror to our deepest shadows. They are our partners in growth and our relationships are a living laboratory where we can examine and begin to heal the parts of us that have been wounded, stunted, and silenced. And being triggered means being uncomfortable. It means having to be resilient and be brave. So yes, these things take effort, but in the same way that going to the Moon or climbing Mount Everest take effort. Those are adventures, not boring slogs, and your relationship effort should feel the same way.

Think about it this way: Out of the 8.1 billion people in the universe, out of all the eras, out of all the countries, out of all the dimensions, you and your partner met here. Perhaps you've even created souls together in your children. That is not happenstance. That is not boring or arduous. That is magic and meaning at your very fingertips. So take a moment and honor how sacred and special that is.

PLEASURE FOR A LIFETIME OF SEX MAGIC

IF YOU'RE FREE AND SINGLE

If you're currently single, take a moment and honor how sacred that is. You have an unwritten epic love story waiting for you to pick up the pen. You have made conscious and subconscious space for the possibility of perfect love, and you will not accept anything less. Again, do you know how rare that is?

To be a conscious, connected, and awakened person is not just a gift, but also a responsibility. I believe that there are a number of us on this planet who are here to be cycle-breakers. People who were born to experience deep trauma and pain, only to rise from the ashes and rebuild new paradigms. We are people who don't want the love we see in Hollywood or on social media. We want love that challenges us and builds us and allows us to redefine what long-term love means.

If you are struggling to find love, you might have a story that you're too old or have too much baggage. Maybe you think all the good ones are taken, or that you missed your chance, or that you're just not desirable enough. Maybe you think the opposite sex can't be trusted and you have deep despair and distrust around dating.

Consider a new story: You're an adventurer who has refused to settle for anything other than the love you desire. You've held yourself during your darkest nights and waited for the one, and in turn they are waiting for you. Your soulmate is out there, seeking you, just as ardently as you are seeking them. You don't have to wait for anything. You don't have to deny yourself anything. Pleasure is yours for the taking. Joy is yours for the taking. You are grateful for every unexpected wave the universe sends you, for you are learning how to steer your ship.

If you ever feel lost on your sex magic journey, just come back to a soft space. Let your body relax, your jaw release, your breath deepen.

And just take a moment to remember that these challenges in your life happen for a reason and that the solutions to these challenges lie within you. Come back to the realization that your partner wants love and desire the same as you do, and that you have the power to bring that to them—and that you have the power to bring that to yourself too. You are the magnet in your relationship, and you can pull whatever you want into your world.

But don't be afraid to ask for help, to seek out like-minded souls who are trying to build a conscious world. Therapy is also invaluable and something every relationship needs—yes, even seemingly perfect ones. Therapy can help deepen your bond and safeguard against future issues. It's not a treatment you use or begin once your relationship is already in trouble. Think of it instead as a preventative measure.

FINAL THOUGHTS

Finally, I leave you with this: Love is something we consciously commit to and something we make anew each day to give to the people around us and to give to our most intimate partners. It is this effort and this conscious intention that make love special.

We get to choose making love new as our primary intention and goal every day. It's not something we have to do. It's the choosing that makes it priceless. It's the choosing that makes it eternal and unending. That we had the choice to be selfish, petty, frightened, or otherwise shut off from love, and we chose instead to bravely commit to being vulnerable and open. That we had the choice to stick with the status quo and accept a mediocre sex life, and instead chose to confront our inhibitions and prioritize passion. The beauty is in the choice. The excitement is in the choice. The choice is pure magic.

ACKNOWLEDGMENTS

I am so grateful for the thirty-plus-year career I have had helping others learn to love and be loved better. I keep thinking I have nothing else to share, and then a new topic inspires me, like sex magic! If it weren't for the amazing clients and students I've been so lucky to work with, I don't know that I would continue to be so inspired. Their open hearts and minds open mine. Their willingness to trust me, and to put their love lives and relationships in my hands, moves me to reverence every time. I am so grateful to BenBella Books for taking a chance on me and this topic I am so passionate about teaching. I am so grateful to Victoria Carmody, Camille Cline, Amy Handy, and the entire BenBella team for their diligent and thoughtful support in bringing this book to fruition. Thank you for being so open-minded and gentle with your edits!

Thank you to Billy Saleeby at Podify for being such a wonderful partner in podcasting and content creation in *Sex Magic* and all things, and to Sam Davidson, Darla Biana, Alex Nguyen, and Muhammad Umar on the Podify team for bringing all my crazy visions to life! Thank you dearly to my literary agent at Paradigm Talent Agency, Ian Kleinert, who was steadfast in finding the right home for *Sex Magic*. I am also so grateful to Bill Douglass for bringing me into

ACKNOWLEDGMENTS

Paradigm and being my constant champion, not to mention his wife, Sahaja, who has become a soul sister and fellow traveler on this and all journeys.

My community of soul friends has seen me through the worst of times and the best of times and have been my rocks, my cheerleaders, and my partners in growth. I am so filled with gratitude that they are in my life. There are more than I can mention here, but just to list those who have kicked my butt or held my hand through the process of writing *Sex Magic*: Hope Ashby, Erika Barrantes, Munisha Bhatia, Tina Cameron, Genevieve Deely, Maria Gonzalez-Terrazas, Susan Grau, Bryan Grijalva, Ann Hoeger, Elyse Klein, Susan Hyman, Lucy Moog, Anita Moorjani, Carter Sharfstein, Bobbi Vogel, Dana Weinstein, Elisabeth Weinstock, Randy Wilder, and Karen Zucker. I love and adore each and every one of you!

To my therapist, healer, and spiritual teacher of seven-plus years, Maureen Riley, thank you for seeing me through the darkest days, and helping me access the wisdom of Source to infuse into this book and everything I do.

To my parents, Linda and Irwin Berman, both no longer on this plane, thank you for teaching me about love. Thank you for loving me so deeply and challenging me to love myself. As I was lucky enough to tell each of you in your final days, thank you for all the ways you wounded me as well, because without those "Big T" and "little t" traumas you bestowed upon me, I never would be the healer I am today. I never would have had the joy and abundance in my life I have achieved from all the healing I have done. It's because of all I've learned from (and as a result of) being your child that I am the clinician I am today, and able to write this book. Your willingness to support my healing and to hold space for my (hard) truths were the most priceless and loving gifts you could give me as parents. I am eternally

ACKNOWLEDGMENTS

grateful. And to my honorary mother, Sandra Flowers, you were love personified, and you were the first one to teach me I was worthy of healing, and to lean into faith.

To my oldest and youngest children, Ethan and Jackson, it has been my greatest joy to watch you grow into the caring, brilliant, powerful, creative and respectful young men you are. I am so grateful I get to be your mama. To my Sweet Boy Sammy, forever sixteen, it is through losing you that I found out how strong I truly am. And it's through the deep longing to stay connected to you that I have opened so deeply to the metaphysical world and discovered all the miracles there. There are more to be found, and while I would do anything to have you back, I am forever grateful for all you continue to teach me.

And to my beloved and eternally patient husband, Sam Chapman, you are my greatest teacher and most favorite companion and cheerleader. You still make my uterus contract after twenty-plus years when I see you walk into a room, and you still make my belly hurt from laughing so hard. Thank you for your steadfast loyalty, your creativity and brilliance, and for being as committed to fueling and sustaining the passion between us as I am. Thank you for letting me change and grow exactly as I need, and for being willing to grow right alongside me.

APPENDIX: SUPPLEMENTAL READINGS

Looking for more information on some of the topics covered in this book? Here, I share some great books on a variety of relevant topics. Enjoy!

CONNECTING TO THE ENERGY WITHIN YOU

Dyer, Dr. Wayne W. *Wishes Fulfilled*. Chapter 9, "Retrain Your Brain So Your Mind Can Work." Hay House, 2013.

Eden, Donna. *Energy Medicine: Balancing Your Body's Energy for Optimal Health, Joy and Vitality*. Jeremy P. Tarcher, 2008.

Kuhn, Greg. *Why Quantum Physicists Do Not Fail: Learn the Secrets of Achieving Almost Anything Your Heart Desires*. CreateSpace Independent Publishing Platform, 2013.

Pert, Candace. *Molecules of Emotion*. Simon & Schuster, 1999.

Williamson, Marianne. *A Return to Love*. HarperOne, 1996.

APPENDIX: SUPPLEMENTAL READINGS

SOMATIC HEALING/EMBODIMENT RESOURCES

Dana, Deb. *Polyvagal Practices: Anchoring the Self in Safety.* W. W. Norton and Company, 2023.

Levine, Peter and Anne Frederick. *Walking the Tiger: Healing Trauma.* North Atlantic Books, 1997.

McConnell, Susan. *Somatic Internal Family Systems Therapy: Awareness, Breath, Resonance, Movement and Touch in Practice.* North Atlantic Books, 2020.

Van der Kolk, Bessel. *The Body Keeps the Score: Brain, Mind, and Body in the Healing of Trauma.* Penguin Books, 2014.

SHIFTING OR IMPROVING THE ENERGY INSIDE YOU AND BETWEEN YOU

Berman, Laura, PhD. *The Book of Love: Every Couple's Guide to Emotional and Sexual Intimacy.* Dorling Kindersley, 2013.

Berman, Laura, PhD. *It's Not Him, It's You!: How to Take Charge of Your Life and Create the Love and Intimacy You Deserve.* Dorling Kindersley, 2011.

Berman, Laura, PhD. *Loving Sex: The Book of Joy and Passion.* Dorling Kindersley, 2011.

Berman, Laura, PhD. *Quantum Love: Use Your Body's Atomic Energy to Create the Love Life You Desire.* Hay House, 2016.

Berman, Laura, PhD. *Real Sex for Real Women.* Dorling Kindersley, 2011.

Berman, Laura, PhD. *You're Not Crazy, You're Just Ascending.* Kindle and Audible e-book, 2021.

APPENDIX: SUPPLEMENTAL READINGS

Brown, Brené. *Atlas of the Heart: Mapping Meaningful Connection and the Language of the Human Experience*. Random House, 2021.

Daedone, Nicole. *Slow Sex: The Art and Craft of Female Orgasm*. Grand Central Life & Style, 2012.

Katie, Byron. *Loving What Is: Four Questions That Can Change Your Life*. Harmony, 2002.

Moorjani, Anita. *Dying to Be Me: My Journey from Cancer to Near Death to True Healing*. Hay House, 2014.

Perry, Dr. Bruce D. *What Happened to You?: Conversations on Trauma, Resilience and Healing*. Flatiron Books, 2021.

SEX SPELLS AND USING SEX FOR MANIFESTATION

Culling, Louis T. *A Manual of Sex Magick*. Llewellyn Publications, 1971.

Frater U∴D∴. *Sex Magic: Release and Control the Power of Your Erotic Potential*. Llewellyn Publications, 2018.

Miller, Jason. *Sex, Sorcery and Spirit: The Secrets of Erotic Magic*. New Page Books, 2014.

Randolph, Paschal, and Maria de Naglowska. *Magia Sexualis: Sexual Practices for Magical Power*. Inner Traditions, 2012.

ABOUT THE AUTHOR

Dr. Laura Berman is a world-renowned sex, love, and relationship therapist. She earned two master's degrees and a PhD from New York University and has spent the past thirty years devoting her career to helping others learn to love and be loved better from a mind, body, and spiritual perspective.

Dr. Berman is a columnist for *USA Today* and a *New York Times* bestselling author who has written nine books. She is also an award-winning syndicated radio host and currently hosts the popular love and sex advice podcast *The Language of Love*.

In addition to her regular appearances in daytime and news media, Dr. Berman was also the sex, love, and relationship expert on *The Oprah Winfrey Show* and has starred in four television series, including two on the OWN Network, one on Showtime, and one on Discovery Network.